Hello, Hello:

The Inspirational Guide to Postpartum

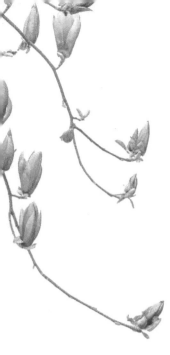

ALSO BY DANIELLE JAI WATSON

HELLO, HELLO:
The Inspirational Guide to Pregnancy

HELLO, HELLO:
The Inspirational Guide to Delivery

www.HelloHelloMom.org

Hello, Hello:

The Inspirational Guide to Postpartum

Danielle Jai Watson

Dedicated To:

Troy and Victoria Boston: the two souls who created the life I have, who never left my side, encouraged me to embrace my power, and allowed me to purpose my dream with extraordinary support — letting me grow and evolve in order to discover the person I dreamed of becoming.

I love you forever, Mom and Dad.

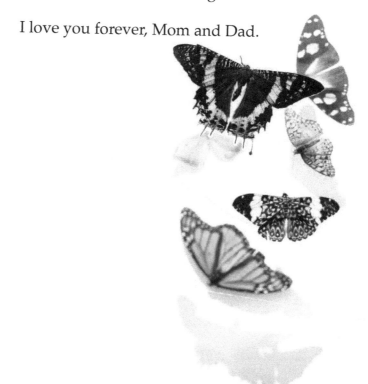

Acknowledgements

Inspired by:

Davi Khalsa, Rashida Cohen, Andrea Custis, Beatrice Dabney, Yodit Crouch, Jasmine Witt, Donna Marshall, Dana Hutchinson, Candace Brown, Quinetta Shaw, Brit'ne Brown, Britney Thomas, Shannon Smith-Holmes, Dnay Baptiste, and my fearless mother in love, Momma Sophie — the powerhouse of women who ignited this journey and made me believe that I was worthy of it. I love you all more than you'll ever know.

In Memory of:

Susie Olive Miles, the one whose fighting spirit lives through me. Mary Etta Dabney Hodge Boston, the one whose passion emanates through everything that I do. And Louise Daniel Hutchinson, my angel who blessed me with the gift and love of all things literary. Your spirit lives on and I will forever be indebted to you. I love you all from now until forever continues.

Made Possible by:

My husband Dion Watson, whose infectious spirit ignites every single space he enters. Thank you for pushing and uplifting me. You see the highest parts of my soul. And to my beautifully kind, brave, and intelligent babies, King Jay and Zenzile Monét Louise Watson — you stripped all the old and poured in the new. The greatest gifts I've ever been given. You make it all make sense.

Written because:

I promised my best friend I would write this book. So I did. I love you Grandad (Ellsworth Hutchinson Jr, WWII Vet).

I hope this makes you proud. Love, Tuffy.

Table of Contents

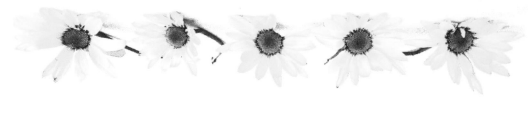

Hello, Hello Beautiful

*I*t is with humble gratitude and an enormous amount of empathy that I offer you my compassion project. With a sole purpose of creating a safe space for you to learn about the task at hand, requiring the grandest amount of human resilience, my desire is to offer the inspiration needed to vitalize an uplifting perspective on motherhood.

With great sensitivity, this book brings forth information about your postpartum care (which I believe is the entire first year). I am not here to convince you of anything other than my belief that you can become exactly who you have always dreamt of becoming — and that you'll indeed make it through every contraction, wave of adversity, and conscious or subconscious fear that may arise.

During my first pregnancy, I was thrust into a whirlwind of emotions. I was so excited — and in the same breath, realized I knew nothing about what I was supposed to do next. In the beginning of my journey, I followed the current traditional path of finding an OB-GYN who would give me tons of ultrasounds, so I could collect the pictures for my future scrapbook.

I arrived to the office and was immediately handed a piece of paper: PLEASE SELECT THE KIND OF DELIVERY YOU DESIRE. I gazed at my husband with a confused look. How was it that in this moment, with my first baby and not even having met a doctor, I could be expected to select a cesarean section (i.e. major surgery)? Why was that even an *option* for me? Still uninformed about what was happening to my body, I continued to follow protocol. I met with the team (there were five different doctors at the office), each instructing me to "… just relax for the next nine months and enjoy eating for two."

Yes, they actually told me to sit down and eat.

Five months into my pregnancy, my aunt, Dr. Rashida Cohen, asked me a question that would lead me to write this book series: *"Have you considered a home birth?"* I wasn't offended by the question. Rather I was upset with myself for still not knowing what was going on with my body, or that there were different options for any number of things — including delivery.

In that moment, I went home and started reading and researching — one of the very things my OB-GYNs had instructed me not to do as to avoid "getting scared by information online."

The more I researched, the more I realized I didn't know much. The more I realized that I'd been willing to do more research on which hair dye I was going to use post delivery —

more so than the technicalities of growing a life within me, and the options I possessed for childbirth.

The more I researched, the more obvious it became to me that most of us have no clue what is going on until we are knee deep in the game. In time, I discovered how embarrassingly high the United States maternal death rate is (the highest among all industrialized countries). The maternal death rate in the U.S. today is WORSE now than it was 25 years ago.

According to a recent study by the Centers for Disease Control and Prevention, it's estimated that approximately 900 women die from giving birth each year in the U.S. There are also roughly 50,000 near-death experiences that occur each year, with over half of those deemed completely preventable..1

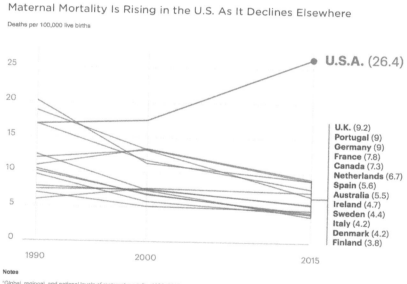

Maternal Mortality Is Rising in the U.S. As It Declines Elsewhere

Deaths per 100,000 live births

Notes

"Global, regional, and national levels of maternal mortality, 1990–2015: a systematic analysis for the Global Burden of Disease Study 2015," *The Lancet.* Only data for 1990, 2000 and 2015 was made available in the journal.

*Graph by NPR Special Series, Lost Mothers: Maternal Mortality In The U.S.*2

The more I read, the more I learned just how often women in the U.S. are subjected to cesarean sections (roughly one out of every three births). Every single one of my peers who'd recently had babies (all under the age of 35 and in exceptional shape as athletes) had cesarean sections. Even with them working out their entire pregnancy, eating healthy and being young, they were all still experiencing the exact same birthing scenarios. How could each woman be having the same problem?

During my research, I learned that medical intervention during delivery has the propensity to cause more harm to a woman's body than actually reducing pain. Even when a woman has never had a baby before, we are more likely to assume that an epidural will somehow make delivery much easier. For some of us, this may be the case. For others, the data seems to suggest otherwise. With roughly 92-94% of women deemed low-risk during pregnancy — or, put another way, 92-94% of women more likely to have a satisfactory birthing experience versus an emergency surgery or some sort of trauma — more than 30% of these healthy women are having major surgery in order to deliver babies (that equals to over 1.2 million women each year in the U.S.).[3]

It became apparent to me that somewhere along the line, mothers have been let down. Interestingly, people were more skeptical of my decision to have both children at home with no medication than they were about a perfectly healthy woman under the age of 35 with no prior medical issues, having major abdominal surgery with opioids and narcotics.

Why was my birthing option deemed less safe when quantifiable evidence shows the opposite?

With home births and hospital births showing no disparity among the infant mortality rate — yet hospital births showing a drastic *increase* in the number of maternal death rates versus home birth, I knew there was something missing for us. And it was, simply: information. Information given in a way that was empathic, nonjudgmental, sensitive, heartfelt and from actual mothers. Whether you decide to birth at home, a birthing center, or hospital, there needs to be a safe space presenting this information in one place, with one goal: to empower!

The more books I found, the more I discovered that *men* are the ones at the head of the ship, deciding the best practices for women during our most vulnerable times. With men never even experiencing a menstrual cramp, let alone understanding the emotional ordeal that a woman experiences through during this journey, I knew it was time to take back our power.

The more videos and documentaries I saw, the more I realized how fearful I was of this entire ordeal. The more I opened my eyes, the more I discovered that everything in my entire life had set me up for a presumption that this would be *the most traumatic experience of my life*. Movies and television shows exemplifying the terror that women face is beyond the pale of necessity: always portraying women as incapable of controlling their minds and emotions during birth; blaming husbands who stand by frantically as if a partner can never be consoling; always rushing into a hospital as if there wasn't a more calming environment in which a woman could bring forth life. I felt manipulated and brainwashed and I knew that others deserved to know every bit of information I'd learned from a place of pure empathy and compassion.Months into my first pregnancy, I knew I had to take the less-traveled road.

Leaving my OB-GYN's office, I met a woman who not only changed my life, but inspired the newest trajectory my life would take. My midwife, Davi Khalsa, gave me information that I knew had to be shared. It had to extend beyond my world and reach those like myself — who are less likely to learn the information and less likely to be sought after. She not only made me feel capable, worthy and strong enough to birth my babies, but she made me feel like I was never alone. She normalized every single feeling I had and that level of personal understanding was something I believe every single woman deserves during this journey.

I knew that my calling was to reach women and reaffirm the power we all inherently possess.

I knew I had to share of my experiences and inspire women to find their own truth and best self during this entire experience — not be told. The judgment that mothers face is extreme and the psychological scar tissue many of us are dealing with (due to traumatic birthing experiences, stress, postpartum care, et cetera) is an underserved topic that has completely taken over my heart. Maternal death rates are staggering. Yet, they can dramatically change. Through education and empowered perspectives on the entire birthing process, we'll begin to take back our power and find comfort in the journey. We will find peace through our education and healing through shared experience.

It is my desire that as you read this book, you find within yourself the resolve to release any fear, guilt or perfectionist ideologies of controlling things outside of your realm. In the same breath, I hope to strengthen your belief in the ability to be powerful right now. It's my goal to encourage you to seek more information on the topics discussed here, in order to best apply them to your life in the most beneficial ways. It is my deepest hope that you never feel judged or bad for any choices you make with your body. This personal journey of motherhood is different for every single woman. And it's my aspiration that I encourage a level of empathy and sensitivity, understanding and care, open-mindedness and curiosity for this most important moment in time.

As a perpetual student of life, it has become increasingly clear to me that people would much rather remain in a state of misinformation, misunderstanding or ignorance toward a topic if made to feel inadequate, insufficient or degraded. I've worked with every breath in my body to ensure you are never made to feel as such.

With care and grave attention to my words, I hope to only embolden curiosity about your body and the wonder you were designed to fabricate. With such a sensitive topic comes a great deal of responsibility and it's something I do not take lightly.

It is with great love that I've created this book in hopes of changing the world in powerful ways. For it's through our knowledge as women that we will become empowered enough to take back our birthright, to birth how we see fit and to survive. It's our responsibility to produce life and keep the universal life-force thriving. And the time is more relevant than ever to get back in the driver's seat of our own birth stories.

I pray you are as inspired by this book as I am by you.

Your beauty, strength, resilience and faith aren't lost on me now, nor will they ever be.

You are a remarkable human being.

You were built for this.

I hope by the end of this read, you'll feel the same way.

With love,

Danielle Jai Watson

"When you love who you are, everything changes."

–Danielle Jai Watson

chapter 1

Hello, Hello Postpartum: Be Inspired

Congratulations mama! You did it! No matter how baby got here; no matter how well you think you did or didn't do; no matter what happened; you did it. You're a superhero! Now that baby is here, making it through one of the toughest moments of your life, real life begins. With each superwoman comes her kryptonite, and we each have one (or two, three, four, or ten). Since we often times solely focus on pregnancy and delivery, the 4th trimester tends to hit us like a ton of bricks.

Postpartum care, aka the 4th trimester, is one of the most vital times for moms. After the initial moment of bliss, the reality of the situation can become so heavy, sudden, and unexpected that we lose ourselves. It seems lonely, and at times feels regrettable. The joy of motherhood is the obvious component, but the true emotions we harbor as women most times go unnoticed, ignored, or blatantly dismissed. Often times, once the baby has arrived, the level of medical care and attention drastically decreases. Aside from healthcare checkups, comes a decrease in familial and friendly checkups. Many people, unless parents themselves, don't realize the weight that comes with this transition. The isolation can become psychologically traumatic, and it's something we all should start to value and focus on — on a gargantuan global level.

The beauty of the 4th trimester comes from the fact that you can still be your best self in your newly evolved space. All hope is not lost. The same manner in which you watch your favorite athletes, musicians, teachers, et cetera, continue their dreams post motherhood, you possess that same strength. You can still become the woman you have always dreamed of — you can still dream (and dream big at that). With the right amount of support, psychological care, self-love and education, anything is possible. And I do mean anything.

Post-delivery, it's imperative once the adrenaline slows down and life starts to kick in, that you find someone (or a group of people) you can talk to about whatever, whenever. During this time, whatever you feel is right. We aren't always right, but we are right to express our feelings.

We're ALL just figuring this thing called motherhood out as we go. There is no one single way to raise our babies. There is no one single way to handle parenting. There is no one way to be a great mother. It simply starts when the unconditional love and resilient investment is there. All we can do is our best. And it's best we recognize that our little bundle of joy is entering into our world — we are not caving into their world. As selfish as it may sound, it's imperative we remember to put ourselves in a space of care and love as well. As easy as it is (and instinctual) to do everything for our baby, it's also almost just as instinctual to forego your needs for the needs of everyone else.

My goal for this book is to encourage your truth to shine, and for you to find healing through your toughest moments. I desire for you to realize you're not alone, and that most of us have felt what you feel (or will soon feel) at one moment or another. My goal is to help prepare you for the moments yet to come, and offer inspiration to guide you through where you are. My hope is that you find your hope and smile again — to encourage your spirit not to feel trapped, and to find what makes you happy.

Your baby will be fine, and it's important to remember that the stronger you are mentally, physically, emotionally and spiritually, the stronger you can be for your family.

This book is about you.

This book was written specifically for you.

With love, I hope you continue to or begin to love yourself again.

You're not lost in motherhood, but rather constantly evolving. And you're made better because of it.

chapter 2

Baby's First Bath: The Gift of Vernix Caseosa

The moment baby is born, all you want to do is hug and kiss them. Either way, it's important to know beforehand that there is no pressing need, or health benefits, to washing baby immediately post-delivery. In hospital settings, it's typically one of the first steps after a baby is born. They check the vitals, show baby to mom and wash them so they're clean in their newborn diaper and adorable hat. With a home birth, midwives typically place the baby immediately onto mom, check their vitals while in mom's arms (as much as physically possible), softly wipe the baby down and place them back in their mother's arms. No bath included.

Though it's now common practice, there are no quantifiable health benefits to baby if immediately washed. In fact, when babies are not washed, they're able to soak up the vast benefits of **vernix caseosa** (the layer that protects the baby's skin from fluids in utero). The waxy and cottage cheese like coating that covers baby when they come out of the birth canal should remain on baby for as long as possible. The comfort of such coating creates many benefits for baby, including:

- **Lubrication:** aids in reducing friction as the baby makes their way through the birth canal — the longer baby is in utero, typically the less vernix caseosa there is on the baby's skin.

- **Antimicrobial Proteins:** the extreme sensitivity of a baby's immune system can be strengthened via breastfeeding and vernix caseosa on the baby's skin — helping to protect the newborn from infection post-delivery due to its antioxidants, anti-infection and anti-inflammatory properties.

- **Regulation of Body Temperature:** since it takes time for baby to regulate their own body temperature, properties in the coating help to stabilize their temperature — baby's body temperate is initially regulated by mom when placed on her chest, illustrating how an initial bath can affect their body's immediate attempt at regulation.

- **Natural Moisturizer:** the coating helps to soften the baby's skin and hair, aiding in reduced dryness and increased moisture.

It's also important to keep in mind: babies are not born dirty. The immediate skin to skin between mom and baby is much more of a necessity. A simple towel rub down of baby can remove enough amniotic fluid, blood and meconium if necessary, without removing the coating and making baby clean enough to hold and kiss. It also is a great moisturizer for babies born with a lot of hair! The longer it's on their little bodies, the better.

listen

to your

heart

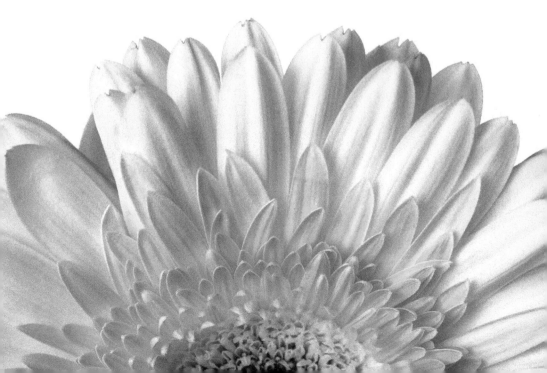

chapter 3

Skin to Skin

Skin to skin is an extremely special and beneficial bonding moment between mom and baby post delivery (and dads too!). Benefits include:

- improvement of heart and lung function as mom's heartbeat can help to calm baby
- stabilization of body temperature
- helps to stabilize blood sugar (helping to combat hypoglycemia in baby)
- aids in breastfeeding (which helps to coat the intestinal wall, boosts digestive function and builds immune system) as baby can find the nipple of choice on their own
- offers good bacteria to baby (when baby passes through the birth canal, the baby's guts are colonized with good bacteria in mom's vagina —

they also continue this colonization of good
bacteria during skin to skin)

- less crying and increased calming of baby

- relief from pain for mom and baby immediately
  post-delivery

- enhancement of mom and baby communication

- reduces stress and makes transition from womb
  easier for baby

- offers a boost in maternal and child bonding

Skin to skin offers many benefits to you and your newborn.
There are times when it may not be a feasible option (i.e. babies
who have to be in NICU, recovering from cesarean section, et
cetera). If you aren't able to practice skin to skin immediately
after delivery, the great news is that the benefits will still parlay
themselves when you get the chance. The moment you finally
get to hold your baby will be just as special. This is not to say
that immediate skin to skin is the only way to create a special
bond post-delivery, but it's one of the most instinctual moments
we tend to have. If you have a hospital birth, it's essential to let
your doctors and nurses know of your desires for immediate
skin to skin. The assumption isn't always made. Stand firm in
your wishes and make it very clear if you want to hold baby
instead of them being rushed into their first bath.

chapter 4

Newborn Shots + Immunizations

Post-delivery, many parents are shocked to discover the number of immediate shots babies are given — and at times, the abrupt nature in which hospital procedures take away a mother's precious first moments with her baby, in order to give newborns shots and tests that can wait. The following lists the immunizations newborns receive (or often receive, depending on the birthing location) in order to help you decide what's best:

- **<u>Apgar Test</u>:** This is the very first test baby will be given as a means to ensure a healthy and successful delivery. Measurements done by midwives and/or nurses are immediate physical assessments focused on their breathing, muscle tone, skin color (they will be checking for the yellow color which can be an early indicator of jaundice, or a blue color to ensure the baby is breathing), heart rate and reflexes/movement. The testing is done on a scale of zero to 10 (10 signifying a healthy baby). Even if baby's number is low initially, studies have shown approximately 98% of babies reach a score of 7 or higher within the first few minutes of life. This will happen quickly and allow you immediate bonding time and skin to skin.

- **Vitamin K:** Most practitioners advise parents to offer this immunization to their newborns. Babies are born with very low levels of vitamin K in their bodies — the vitamin needed in order for blood to clot (i.e. if a baby were to get a cut, without vitamin K, their bodies would have no way to stop the bleeding). There are options for the supplement including a shot (typically done in the thigh) or via liquid oral dosages. Babies who receive the shot will do so just once and many times can be comforted by moms cuddle or breastfeeding soon thereafter. For those who receive the vitamin in oral doses, they will have to do so multiple times in order to complete the dosage. This tends to be a low risk, low side effect, process. Be sure to check with your doctor or midwife to explore all options.

- **PKU (Metabolic Screening):** This is a sample of blood drawn from your newborn's heel that will check for abnormalities in which the baby's body cannot breakdown amino acids found in protein.

Essentially the blood work will screen for up to 30 different diseases that are blind to the naked eye; which could aid in the prevention of problems such as developmental disabilities, brain damage, organ damage, or death. It's important to know what baby is being screened for—something you can find out prior to delivery. This test can occur after initial skin to skin bonding time.

- **Hearing Test**: In many hospitals, a successful newborn hearing test is required prior to being released. This pain free test will check for a baby's hearing (or possible impairments). For those who have home births, your midwife will provide you with a written referral, whereby you'll take baby within the first month to see a hearing specialist who will provide the hearing test. Benefits include finding hearing impairments early in order to help prevent developmental delays and struggles (i.e. speech and language difficulty).

- **Hepatitis B:** This is an extremely important test for mothers who are infected with Hepatitis B. If passed on to a baby who is not properly treated, they become more at risk to develop liver cancer, cirrhosis (chronic liver damage), or death. For those who have tested negative for Hep B, it has been described as a "topic of debate", if it's necessary for your newborn. Essentially, depending on who you are, your belief system

---

and the manner by which (and from whom) you receive this information, your decision on the Hep B vaccination will be entirely up to you. This is not a law-binding vaccine and you should never be forced or made to feel insignificant if you so choose against it. It's important to research the proposed benefits of said vaccination prior to your delivery.

- **<u>Eye Drops (Erythromycin)</u>:** Many hospitals offer (or most times assume) you'll want this for baby. It's essential to research the benefits (or lack thereof) of eye drops for your newborn. Essentially, the drops or ointment are used to help prevent eye infections that can lead to blindness, when mom delivers while having a sexually transmitted infection (most notably chlamydia or gonorrhea). For many moms, the tests taken during prenatal visits will indicate if you have an STI or not. For those who do not, this treatment may be unnecessary for baby. Research and discover what's best for you. This is not bound by law and you should never be pressured into having this done to your baby if you choose not to.

Every birth story is different, as is every delivery and every baby. It's essential for parents to take back the control we have over the initial foundations set for our precious newborns. No single person should be able to tell us what's right or wrong for our children without our knowledge of the information. It's imperative to learn, prior to delivery, what can and should happen in the immediate moments after birth. It's crucial to learn what's needed right away and what can wait — what is imperative for our baby's health and what has become simple routine. The more we know, the better equipped we can be.

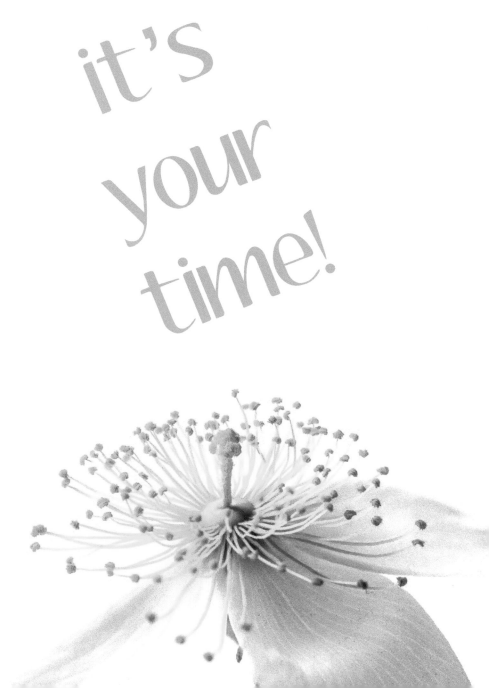

it's
your
time!

chapter 5

Finding the Right Pediatrician

*T*ypically, if all is well with you and baby, your newborn will likely see a pediatrician for their first checkup two or three days after birth. Being that, in those initial days, there is a ton of physical healing, emotional and mental adjustments and a huge leap into a massive learning curve, it may become extremely difficult to search for and find a new pediatrician as well during that time. It's wise to search for a pediatrician about one to two months prior to the due date of delivery, if you have the ability to do so.

This offers you time to explore different pediatricians, ask as many questions as you have and find the best fit for your needs. There are those who are more traditional and vaccine/medication centered, while other practices offer a more homeopathic, less medicinal based practice. There are also pediatricians who fall right in the middle of the spectrum; thus, stressing the importance of finding who works best prior to your delivery.

Spending time with other moms, researching online and setting up appointments (informal interviews) can help ease the difficulty of the process. The beauty is that you can always switch. If a doctor works in the beginning, but through time doesn't meet your needs, then switch. No parent is tied or obligated to stay with a doctor who does not vibrate at the same frequency or meet the demands they require for their children.

Follow your mommy gut and always choose what works best for you and your family. With the advent of a strong technological presence in the medical field, many pediatricians are offering services whereby parents can send texts/images with their medical concerns without having to physically come in to the office space. Some insurance companies also offer "doctor on demand" where you can video chat in real time for immediate consultation. There is a pediatrician out there who can meet your needs. With a little research and time, you'll find the right one.

After your newborn's initial visit, they will likely see their pediatrician at each major milestone. These often include, but are not limited to, six weeks, three months, six months, 9 months and one year. Pediatricians offer varied suggested vaccination timelines, so it's best to learn what those are in the beginning — as the best prepare and make decisions for your family. Your beliefs about vaccinations are for you to uphold. Follow your intuition and remain diligent in your research. Don't be swayed by public opinion or misinformation on either side of the spectrum. You'll know what's best. You got this.

chapter 6

Circumcision: Relieving the Pressure

*T*oo often we as parents are ridiculed into making decisions for our babies. Circumcision is one of those topics and it has become a breeding ground of judgment and insensitivity. The following chapter is not designed in any way to persuade, convince, or encourage a decision for your baby boy. I don't believe there is one right way to care for every baby and it's up to us as parents to decide what we believe will give them the best start in life.

The following information on circumcision is merely offering insight and knowledge on a topic that has often become taboo and/or standard practice without the necessary research. This is simply to start the dialogue and offer information in a manner that will encourage further research (should you deem it necessary) and help alleviate the notion of circumcisions being a topic worth avoiding or coerced into.

For starters, placing the topic in a more cultural world view, most parents around the world are not given the option of circumcising their children "just because". Typically, it's done due to religious beliefs or cultural traditions (and that includes both males and females). Though we often do not consider our baby girls being circumcised, it happens in various parts of the world.

While some may consider circumcision of baby girls as mutilation, the fact that boys and girls are viewed differently in their genital hygiene and immediate needs is simply a cultural norm. For those who practice circumcision for religious beliefs, the topic is a pretty basic one. For those who have no such religious binding traditions, it's simply a matter of personal preference.

In Western practice, the origin of male circumcision started roughly 100 years ago. The belief was that if a boy was circumcised, he would be less likely to masturbate; thus, reducing his sexual desires. There was also a belief that by surgically removing the foreskin of young boys, it would help to significantly reduce a grave number of genital diseases or infections. Through time, as medical research continues to illustrate the lack of benefits from circumcision, more parents are deciding against the surgical procedure (with numbers steadily dropping).

The U.S. is essentially one of the only countries in the world that routinely surgically removes a baby boy's foreskin for non-religious and non-medical reasons. Though many parents are assumed to want the procedure, most of us are not fully informed on the lack of medical benefits the procedure offers. Most of us are also completely unaware of what the surgical procedure entails.

For starters, it's important for us to remember: boys were not born with a foreskin by accident. The simple fact that males and females are born with foreskin, often increases speculation of the need to remove a part of the human body for no medical reason. For most procedures, **prophylactic procedures are done over therapeutic procedures**. According to an article published by the International Childbirth Education Association:

> "...almost all circumcisions in the U.S. are performed to prevent a possible future problem, that is, for prophylactic reasons. Such thinking is reminiscent of the prophylactic tonsillectomies recommended for most children a generation ago. When it became obvious that the risks exceeded the benefits, physicians rejected the procedure."[4]

Rather than treating problems, most babies are enduring these surgeries for problems that most likely will not arise in the future otherwise. Herein lies the moment when parents must decide if the proposed risks of the procedure outweigh avoiding the procedure. If it's likely nothing bad will happen to my baby boy if I avoid the surgery, is it really worth the risk of doing it in the first place? For some the answer may be yes, for others no. No matter the answer you choose, that is the right answer for you.

When making the decision, it's important to learn of the importance of infant **smegma**. Researchers used to believe smegma (the secretion found under the foreskin) caused cancer.

This has been completely disproven. Newer research has discovered that not only does smegma not cause cancer, but it's beneficial to the genital area in that it provides a protective coating (natural lubrication for the area).

The **foreskin,** which is removed during circumcision, is also another protective layer designed to aid in genital function. The rounded part at the end of a male's penis and the woman's clitoris is an extremely sensitive area. The foreskin (on both males and females) helps to shield the areas from irritations caused by urine and feces. The foreskin, from infant-hood until adulthood, is there to protect the sensitive glans from infection and irritation. The foreskin also aids in lubricating the glans, helping to stimulate sexual pleasure rather than eliminating sensations or causing premature ejaculation (a claim with no sound basis or proof). With good hygiene (which is equivalent to good hygiene of circumcised genitalia), babies will be just as protected from infections and diseases either way. Keeping clean is essential for all babies; hence, there is no elaborate way to clean an uncircumcised penis of your newborn baby.

Overtime, the foreskin of the uncircumcised penis will retract on its own. The foreskin is typically attached to the glans at birth and through time will retract without the need of it being manually retracted. When doctors tell parents to forcefully retract the foreskin prematurely, it does more damage than good. Doing so will be extremely painful to your newborn and has the potential of causing damage to the surface of the glans underneath the foreskin (which could lead to bleeding and possible infection). Every baby is different — with some being able to having their foreskin retracted within weeks and others taking years. Either way, no harm will come from leaving it alone. The manner by which we leave our girls foreskin alone applies to our boys as well.

For some parents, there has been a line of reasoning for circumcision being that boys will want to look like their fathers. The truth of the matter is that, every child will look different from their parents in some form or fashion. There is no medical evidence a boy will suffer from psychological trauma if his penis looks slightly different than his father's. Children are a product of the manner in which they're raised. If they're raised to feel confident in the skin they're in, they will more than likely believe the same about themselves. The mind is a powerful tool and it's especially vital in the development of open-minded, empathic, kind and compassionate children. They will believe what we tell them. The more power and truth they receive, the stronger they will become.

Whether you decide for or against the surgical procedure, is completely up to you. No one should judge your decision and frankly, no one needs to know. You don't owe anyone a defense of your choice. If you do decide on the surgery, it's essential to learn what methods will occur in the procedure of your precious baby boy. Many hospitals place the baby in a form of restraint, clean the penis, use a probe to forcefully separate the foreskin from the penis, retract it and then use various methods to remove the skin. It's important to remember: babies do feel pain. The notion of them being too young to remember the pain is valid, but still hard to deal with as a parent watching baby endure such pain (some arguing unnecessarily).

Find what speaks to you and learn what your rights. Understand your power in the final decision. Feel empowered in your choice, regardless of what you decide. Refuse to allow yourself to become persuaded by outside opinion. Do what feels right for you and your child. Follow your mommy gut. More often than not, you'll know exactly what to do.

trust yourself

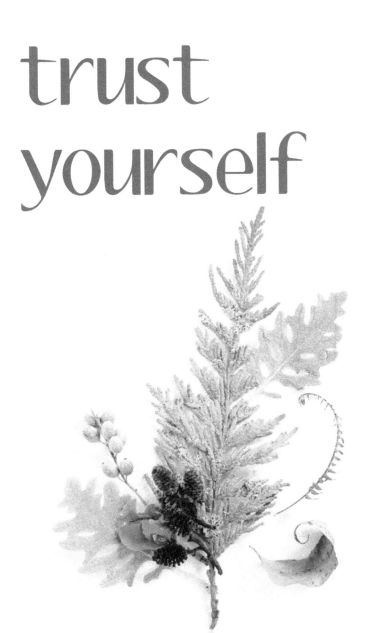

chapter 7

The Umbilical Cord

*U*nless you've seen a newborn baby before, or have had a baby in the past, it may come as a surprise to find that (for most babies) part of the umbilical cord will be left on their belly for a couple of weeks post-delivery. When the umbilical cord is clipped, a clamp is placed on the piece connected to baby's belly. This piece will eventually dry up and fall off — but not for a couple of days, or weeks (about one to four weeks). It's nothing to worry about and will fall off on its own, but it can definitely be an interesting sight if you aren't expecting it. According to the ever-popular site What to Expect, the following lists the best care[5]:

> 1. *Keep it clean*
>
> 2. *Keep it dry*
>
> 3. *Stick to sponge baths*
>
> 4. *Diaper delicately*

5. Dress delicately

6. Resist removing

You'll typically be instructed to steer clear of the cord until it falls off naturally. You won't need to wash it or pull on it (even if it looks to be hanging on by a thread). The dryer it stays, the faster it will heal and fall off. You'll want to be careful as not to snag it in the diapers or while changing clothes and you'll need to ensure there aren't any signs of infection which include (as listed by *What to Expect*):

- *red or swollen*

- *fluid filled lump near the cord*

- *oozing of pus (or any foul-smelling discharge)*

- *bleeding (a little dried blood is normal)*

- *fever, lethargy, low appetite, irritability*

- *abdominal swelling*

With care and precaution, most babies will sail through this short phase with ease. The less you stress over it, the easier the process. The less you bother it, the better it will be. Simple enough.

chapter 8

Jaundice

A very common (and often self-correcting) condition newborns face is **jaundice**. It's apparent by the yellowing of a baby's skin or eyes — an indication that the newborn's liver hasn't matured enough to secrete bilirubin through the digestive tract. **Bilirubin** creates a process that clears the body of aged red blood cells through our waste system. Time and proper feeding of baby typically allows it to pass on its own (usually by three weeks old).

Fortunately, checking for jaundice in newborns is a routine process prior to being released from the hospital and post-delivery of home births. Midwives who continue to check on mom at home in the days and weeks after giving birth, also check for jaundice in baby — as well as baby's pediatrician. As most circumstances result in self correction, there are times when it doesn't and a baby needs to be checked for more underlying conditions.

It's best to focus on the well-being of baby and take it day by day. Feeding baby on demand (if possible) can help to ensure they're receiving the nutrients needed as their liver matures — helping to pass the bilirubin through their system. Premature babies, those who have a different blood type then their mom and those who aren't receiving enough milk (possibly due to feeding difficulties), are at a higher risk of developing jaundice.

If you're struggling with breastfeeding, it's important to share that information with your doctor, midwife, lactation specialist, and/or pediatrician. There are options (i.e. organic formula, breastmilk donation, et cetera) to help you overcome this hurdle. Many women find that using other mothers' breastmilk as a supplement until their own milk comes in and as feedings get better and easier, helps to keep their baby on the right track of exclusive breastfeeding (avoiding the use of formula). Sometimes formula may be the thing you need.

If the jaundice doesn't pass, specialty treatments will aid in breaking down and passing the bilirubin from your newborn's body. One popular treatment includes **phototherapy**. This is a light treatment in which the newborn is placed on a special bed with protective goggles. The light aids in removing the bilirubin from the body. Typically, after a few days or less, the baby's body will regulate and have safe levels of the chemical in their body. With side effects usually including diarrhea, dehydration or skin irritations, this is manageable in comparison to the side of effects of unchecked bilirubin levels (which could include bilirubin making its way to the newborn's brain).

With such effective means of reversing and correcting this condition, it's important to keep in mind the normality of mild jaundice appearing in the early days/weeks of life and the high probability that all will be well. In some severe cases, a blood transfusion may be necessary. Try not to stress, as stress inhibits the success of breastfeeding and reduces milk supply. Relax and breathe. Everything will be alright (tell yourself this as much as you need to). It will.

baby chose you for a reason

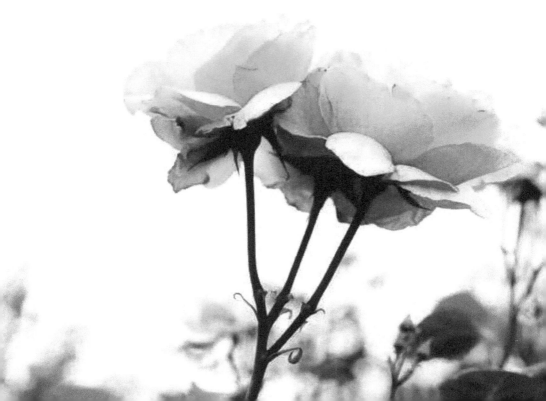

chapter 9

Mom's Immediate Needs

Per the usual motions post-delivery, most attention will be on your newborn. In more personal settings such as home births, it may feel less isolating as the attention is on both mom and baby equally. In hospitals, there are rules and traditions whereby standards move from baby first to mom second. The efficiency of hospital practices has drastically decreased the likelihood of infant mortality, so it's not something to take lightly. Yet in the same breath, it's well understood when talking with mothers who birth in hospitals, just how isolating that special moment often becomes as all the attention goes immediately to the baby (at times leaving the mother out of the very moment).

Your own instincts will also place the needs of baby first (it's nature's way). But it's essential to be aware that you too have pressing and immediate needs as well. If you, mom, aren't well, then the foundation to the start of this new journey is more likely to be harder and more stressful. It's imperative to find those with whom you can communicate how important it will be to have help and attention immediately post-delivery and during the weeks and months to come.

Though it's more likely for postpartum needs to come as a shock to the system, it's my hope that this chapter helps to shed light on how the first couple of weeks will go (things that aren't often mentioned until we are thrust into the moment).

Your First Pee

Your first pee (and possible subsequent trips to the bathroom — sometimes for weeks) will probably hurt! The very first pee can be somewhat scary, especially having just pushed a baby out. There are many reasons for pain and/or irritation while using the bathroom after delivery. Some include:

- swelling
- tears (whether stitches were needed or not)
- trauma (i.e. if a catheter was used for cesarean section)
- or possible urinary tract infections

For roughly 90% of moms, we will experience some sort of swelling or damage in the vaginal area — resulting in painful urination. Unfortunately, there isn't much relief you can find for the very first trip to the bathroom. You'll just have to do it (and you can because you're strong)! It's also essential you pee within the first few hours after giving birth to avoid having a full bladder. A **full bladder** post-delivery can result in bleeding, damage, or infection to the bladder. The following sections share some ways to help ease or alleviate the pain you may experience and hopefully will encourage to allow yourself time to fully heal.

The Squirt Bottle

Hospitals and home births will ensure you have a squirt bottle to use after delivery. Essentially, you'll want to have warm (not hot) water in the bottle to squirt on your vagina and/or perineum with every urination. This helps to ease the area that is sensitive and aids in keeping it as clean as possible. You'll likely use this while you pee and again after you finish, prior to putting on your really large pad (from the heavy bleeding). You'll also likely use the restroom a lot as you ensure personal hydration (especially if breastfeeding, as its imperative to stay hydrated for milk production and strong health).

Witch Hazel Pads

You'll also need to use witch hazel pads to clean the area after each time in the restroom. This can help provide cooling relief to possible tears and/or swelling and aid in reducing inflammation caused by hemorrhoids. You could also freeze some regular menstrual pads to place on top of your sanitary pads to help provide cooling and healing properties to your vagina. Your doctor or midwife may also offer lidocaine ointment or spray to help ease the pain (ask about your options).

Ice For Your Vagina

Ice packs placed directly on your vagina will be your very best friend for the first couple of days. With most women experiencing swelling post vaginal delivery, the ice will feel incredibly awesome and aid in reducing inflammation. You can make the perfect ice packs right at home before you deliver. A week or so prior to your due date, take about 12 heavy flow pads out of the wrapper and dip them in a bowl of water. Let out a little of the water as not to have it completely soaked — but it should be sufficiently wet. Then place the wet sanitary pads in a large plastic freezer bag and place in the freezer. Post-delivery (for home births) you'll have the perfectly suited ice pack that can also absorb your bleeding. This ice pack will go on top of your dry, heavy flow pad — allowing them to fit seamlessly one on top of the other. If you have a hospital birth, your nurses will offer you some sort of ice relief on site.

Once home, you'll have your own ice packs in case swelling and irritation persists. Remember that optimum pushing positions can help to significantly reduce the amount of swelling and likelihood of tearing, as discussed in *Hello, Hello: The Inspirational Guide to Delivery.*

Pelvic Weakness

As to be expected, a lot of pressure occurs to your pelvic floor during the pregnancy and birthing process. The hormone relaxin, pressure on your bladder from the baby's weight and pushing (or use of medical interventions such as forceps during delivery), can cause stress to the pelvic floor — thus, weakening those muscles. For some women, these weakened muscles result in leaking (explained in more detail in the *Pelvic Weakness/ Incontinence* chapter). Others include having strong urges to use the restroom but having the inability to do so. This may be caused by a urinary tract infection (which is more likely to occur with use of epidurals or catheters).

And then there are those who cannot use the restroom at all (known as postpartum urinary retention). This may be the result of an untreated urinary tract infection, or the result of numbing of the bladder caused by the epidural medication. The importance of relieving your bladder within the first couple of hours after delivery is essential in helping to avoid the bladder becoming too full and becoming infected. Try to relax and breathe the first pee out. Be open and honest if you're suffering in this way.

Hemorrhoids

There are times when the stress and/or strain of pushing can result in hemorrhoids. *(Note: Optimal pushing positions and reduced use of medical numbing intervention can help to minimize weakened pushing and increase your chances of working with gravity to deliver).* The use of witch hazel pads as well as soaking in your sitz bath can be a great help in relieving the pain. Avoid sitting on your bottom for prolonged periods of time, as that can aggravate the area. By resting and taking it easy during your immediate healing process, it should heal within six weeks or so. Remember, each body is different. Take everything at your own pace.

Vaginal Bleeding

You may (or may not) have heard of the postpartum period. For the next 4-6 weeks, your body will be flushing out **lochia** which is a combination of blood, mucous and tissue from your uterus, to be released from your vagina (cue the need for extremely absorbent pads). As the weeks progress, your bleeding will begin to taper. It will be reminiscent of a normal to heavy period, as your body sheds of the remaining tissue from your uterus. It's important to monitor your flow — as not to continuously soak through your pads (which could be the sign of an infection). It's also important to monitor the size of blood clots that may pass through as well. It may be terrifying to see a ball of blood literally plop of your vagina, but it's normal and healthy. If, though, your blood clot is the size of a softball or bigger, it's time to notify your doctor or midwife — as this too could be a sign of a possible infection. If and when the ball of blood falls out that isn't too big, don't panic. Everything is okay (it's just weird).

Emptying Your Bladder Before Nursing

As previously noted, it's essential to empty your bladder within the first couple of hours post- delivery to avoid over stretching the bladder, which could lead to bleeding and/or infection. Emptying your bladder often can help to allow for your pelvic muscles to heal (avoiding expansive stretching which puts pressure on the bladder). It's also important to use the restroom prior to nursing to avoid an expanding bladder. As you nurse, you'll likely become dehydrated and need to drink more. Drinking more requires releasing more. Within the first few weeks or months of breastfeeding (as your milk begins to relegate), you'll likely drink while you nurse to help avoid dehydration (which can also lead to cramping). Release yourself before you nurse, to help keep your bladder from overworking.

Give Yourself Time

It seems more intuitive to move slowly post a cesarean section, as most times you physically aren't capable of abrupt movements. With vaginal delivery (especially if done without medical intervention), your body gets a full and large dose of adrenaline and oxytocin. This may cause you to feel extremely strong and ready to take on the world. It's important, though, for the next couple of weeks to get up and out of bed with a bit more patience to help avoid moving too fast — causing you to get dizzy. It's also important to keep in mind your fluctuating hormones during this time. This could lead to postpartum vertigo, dizziness, or migraines. Take it easy and listen to your body.

Keeping Your Maternity Clothes (just for a while)

As you know, the hormone relaxin released throughout the body during pregnancy aids in the relaxing of muscles and ligaments, to allow for your growing baby (as noted in *Hello, Hello: The Inspirational Guide to Pregnancy*). It also allows your hips to widen to make space for your beautiful baby to push through. There are often times when mom's hips are a little bit wider for good. This is okay and does not signify a problem.

Due to your newly enhanced goddess body, you may still find it difficult to fit into your pre-pregnancy jeans — even if you have lost all of the pregnancy weight.

During the first few weeks/months, your maternity apparel may be extremely comfortable as you recover and adjust to your new normal. It's important, though, to eventually rid of the maternity gear. You won't need them forever, even if they're your go-to. Our goal is not to create a habit of wearing maternity clothes — yet receive the benefits of their comfort in the early days. Eventually, we will need to get out of the pregnancy gear in order to bring about a sense of normalcy, a simple nod to your past, and an acceptance of the newly evolved (and sexy) person you are becoming.

Nutrition and Exercise

In most countries around the world, postpartum care for mothers is a priority — most often including a small window of time dedicated to "confining" mom and baby. Family and friends take care of the essentials, while mom heals and bonds with baby in a relaxed setting. This is not the norm in Western cultures, where the art of moving fast and always having to get things done reigns supreme. Because of this reality, nutrition can be hard to focus on and come by as a new mom. Whereby others may have family members cooking meals with proper nutrition for them, many moms today are forced to make a choice: sleep or make time for a well balanced diet (sleep always wins by the way). This is why it is important to find help and make it a point to focus on your personal nutrition — in the same manner that you do for your baby.

You too need the same (if not more) care when it comes to postpartum nutrition in that, it is the way in which you heal and provide food for your baby. You will need nutrient rich and dense foods to help aid and strengthen your body as it heals (and as it releases nutrients for you baby via nursing). What we eat or don't eat will effect our mood. The stronger our choices, the stronger and more energized we will feel. We are what we eat, and it is extremely hard to eat right with a newborn and little help. Make this a priority because you are the priority.

After you have allowed your body the initial healing time (typically 6 weeks, but complete healing can take upwards of 12 months), start your workouts slowly. Again, there is no rush. If you jump in too quickly, it will take your body even longer to heal internally - even if you are losing weight. Start with walking, and find creative ways to workout with your baby. Also, find ways to exercise without your baby. You will need alone time and personal downtime. This is important for your sanity and rejuvenating your spirit. Make it a part of your priority list. You will thank yourself soon thereafter.

Vitamins and Medication

You'll want to take your pain medication and vitamins (i.e. ibuprofen, DHA, calcium, magnesium, et cetera), to help alleviate the pains of childbirth and rejuvenate your body. Incorporating supplements into your new routine can drastically impact your ability to function within the first couple of weeks and months. Taking your medication regularly for the first few days may have you feeling back to normal. Without them, your abdomen will remind you of just how strenuous labor was.

NOTE: Ibuprofen may also help with abdominal pain while driving. The stress of labor on your abs makes it very hard to engage those muscles for everyday tasks, including driving. Take it slow.

Take what you need and do what you need in order to feel your best. The better you feel, the better you can be for yourself and baby. Vitamins are also essential to your well-being— helping to fill your body with extra nutrients that you may be missing from your diet (and those depleted through nursing). In the upcoming chapter, a list of vitamins is provided that will be extremely beneficial to your overall healing and well-being.

Your First Poop

It's important to remember your stool softener. Most doctors and midwives will add stool softener to your postpartum routine. This is essential in your overall well-being. Post-delivery, your body takes time to readjust to your now pregnancy free body (i.e. free from the high levels of relaxin that caused your digestive tract to significantly slow down). This can cause constipation — alongside exhaustion from sleep deprivation and the struggle for a well-balanced diet. Stool softeners will help move the stool along without the need for serious pushing.

Also, the first poop can be terrifying! For many moms, the first time feels like you're literally going to push your vagina out of your body. It's scary, especially with the high level of sensitivity and awareness to your body. There are some moms who don't have their first bowel movements for three to four days post-delivery. It may be scary, but the more you hold it in the harder it will be to pass. A tip that may help: **hold your vagina**. The sensation of holding your vagina in place may help to alleviate the fears of pushing during your poop. Once it's time to go during your postpartum recovery, nothing will be weird or off limits.

Note: Avoid becoming dehydrated—the more water you drink, the better your chances of alleviating constipation.

Cramping (postpartum contractions)

Immediately after you deliver your baby and placenta, your doctor, nurse, or midwife will **aggressively push on your belly** as a means to initiate the contraction of your uterus. These contractions (though painful and uncomfortable) are essential in ensuring that you don't hemorrhage. Contractions are a good sign your uterus is returning to its pre-pregnancy size. This often comes as a shock to the system for moms — labor is behind us, but we're still experiencing contractions! Fortunately, the pain level is nowhere near your labor contractions, but the cramping may continue for a few weeks post-delivery. Being dehydrated also contributes to cramping, so drink tons of water. Breastfeeding, in the early weeks, can contribute to cramping sensations, as your uterus is doing extra work in shrinking back to its normal size (hence, why women who nurse tend to see their uterus shrink back faster). The good news is that the cramping is only seasonal. In a few weeks, you'll be cramp free.

Vaginal Dryness

You will be dry. The sudden and drastic drop in estrogen (coupled with nursing) causes your vaginal mucosa to thin. When it's time to return to sex in a couple of weeks, you'll need lubrication. Investing in natural oils and lubricants will be essential in protecting your vagina and ensuring great (and comfortable) sex. The longer you breastfeed, the longer you'll need help with dryness. Don't be ashamed about it. It's all about feeling your best. Treat your vagina with care. It's vital. It's the life source. Honor her and honor your need to feel exceptional.

Rest

The most important thing to focus on in terms of postpartum self-care is rest. It's essential you allow your body the time it needs to recover from the most intense and strenuous thing you've ever done with it. If there were no pain killers and ways to ease discomfort, we all would feel like we were hit by a trailer truck 1000 times. We must never degrade the level of intensity that just took place. For the first two weeks, it's imperative you allow yourself the time to just rest. Have help (if you can) with simple things. Don't feel like a burden or as if you're being lazy. Soon enough, you'll never have time to sit down (let alone lay in bed). Take this short window of time for granted. Your body needs to heal, especially while organs are moving back into place.

With adrenaline at an all-time high, you may even feel like you could run a mile. But don't! There is no need. Soon enough you'll be up running around all day and night! Let others do your chores, relax as much as you can, ask for help and be open to receiving it within these first couple of weeks. You need this the same way baby needs you. The better the start, the better the journey.

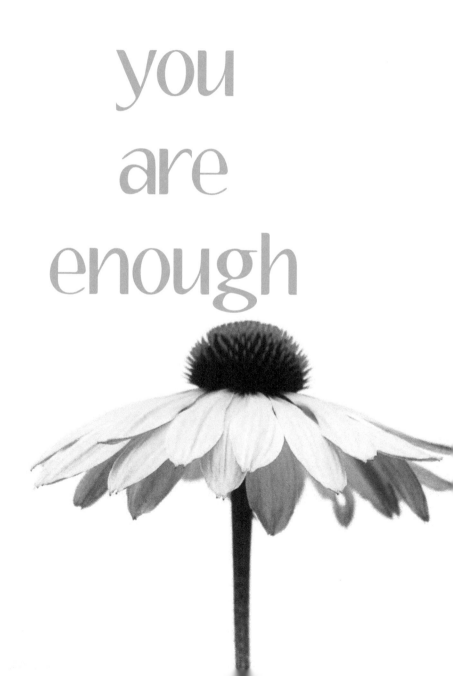

you

are

enough

chapter 10

Visitors (and when to say no)

As mentioned above, rest is essential to your healing and well-being. Rest aids in healing physically, mentally, and emotionally. Aside from physically resting in bed as your body begins to recover, the notion of mental exertion can be daunting as well. This often times comes in the form of visitors and the need to entertain them.

People love to visit babies as soon as they can. It's such a special moment. Yet, even when the best intentions are present, it's imperative to monitor the amount of exhaustion (conscious or subconscious) this causes you. In the early days/weeks, visitors include a ton of labor and delivery storytelling, watching to make sure baby is held properly and is comfortable, making sure people wash their hands constantly, use burp cloths, don't have a cough and so forth. The amount of attention that goes into watching your guest with your very precious newborn is innate and exhausting.

The point: if you're not in the mood for visitors, just say no! Period. If you're exhausted and just don't want to see anyone, just say no. You owe no-one an explanation on how you feel and what you want in this time of your life. You have made it through an intense feat and your feelings are one of the greatest indicators of what you need and what you need to avoid. You can easily become overwhelmed with visitors and people often are so enamored with your newborn they forget about how you feel and what you may need (missing obvious clues regarding your state of being).

A helpful tip is to make clear, prior to delivery, that you'll let people know when you're ready to have visitors. Keep it simple. Follow your mommy gut, listen to your body and mind your spirit. If it doesn't feel right, don't do it. Eventually, you'll need some visitors. This will help to break up the monotonous routine you have just fell in to; it will help give you adult conversation and allow your mind the ability to drift somewhere beyond just a sleeping, eating and pooping baby; and it will allow you time to do something normal (i.e. take a hot shower and wash your hair). But you must do this when you're ready. Even if people feel like they're helping, it may feel like more work for you.

Be honest about what you need and how you feel. Don't apologize for how you feel or the schedule you have set. If you don't want people over at night, don't allow it. If your window of time doesn't work with another's schedule, only adjust should you feel the energy to do so. Remember, you have just delivered a baby. At the end of the day, you and your spouse/

partner are the only ones who will be with baby at all times. When people leave and go about their day / night, you'll be the one up with a colicky baby, or trying to figure out how to nurse, et cetera. Do what you need. Mind your priorities. Make yourself just as important as your new baby. You need it and you deserve it.

fall in love with you

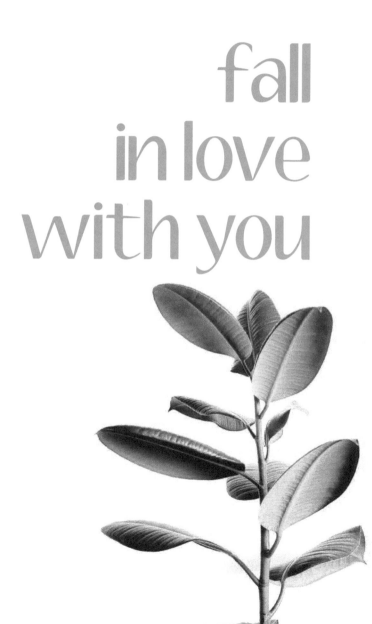

chapter 11

Breastfeeding

One of the most nuanced topics centered around the start of motherhood is breastfeeding. Many of us have heard crazy stories; from it being extremely easy (moms who had so much milk and nursed for three years trouble free), to the horror stories (moms with cracked nipples, would could never produce enough milk and constantly developed mastitis). The truth of the matter is that, no single experience with breastfeeding is the same — yet, you're never alone in whatever you experience.

Every mother struggles, to some degree, with nursing. A mom who seemingly has it easy with nursing may be struggling to wean her 18-month old (no easy feat), while a mother who had a tumultuous start may have made it to three months and felt it necessary to transition to bottle feeding (also not an easy feat). Whatever the case, your journey is yours. It's about doing what's best for baby and your sanity. Though breastmilk is the absolute best vaccine we can provide our newborns, it almost becomes counterproductive if the act itself is done with disdain, resentment, or unbearable pain. Some moms simply can't do it and, if that is you, remember that it's okay. Your baby will be just fine. No judgment. No stress.

This chapter is purely intended to highlight what occurs to your body during milk production, to share some things you can expect (tips to help with pain management) and to explore one manner in which to feed your baby. It's imperative to keep in mind that how you mentally enter into your new journey (how you set the foundation) can most certainly come to fruition. If you go into your breastfeeding journey with negative feelings, it will be a negative experience. If you enter with an empowered outlook (which is inclusive of the realities of inherent struggles), you'll have an empowered experience, you'll nurse for as long as you desire and you'll overcome the adversities of this most precious phase of new motherhood.

The Beginnings

During your pregnancy, you may notice some dried milk on your nipples. Some moms will see evidence of the start of milk production weeks or even months prior to delivery, while others don't notice any significant change until after the placenta is delivered. As noted by Breastfeeding Support:

> *"After the birth of your baby, the placenta separates from the uterus and is expelled. This causes a sharp drop in the hormone progesterone which triggers the breasts to*

start milk production about 32-40 hours after birth. Other important hormones that are needed for milk production are prolactin, insulin and cortisol (stress hormone). Oxytocin is another hormone that triggers the let down of milk at each feed."[6]

Prolactin is the primary hormone your body needs in order to produce milk. During pregnancy, your body has a surge in estrogen and progesterone — both which prevent higher levels of prolactin to be produced throughout your body. Though the levels of prolactin are low, it's still present during pregnancy as it's preparing your breasts to produce mature milk. Once you deliver baby and your placenta, the levels of estrogen and progesterone decrease, allowing your levels of prolactin to significantly increase. This surge of prolactin then initiates the start of your mature milk supply, often leading to engorgement (since your colostrum is now transitioning to mature milk in large amounts) and remains higher than normal for the duration of your nursing experience.

Insulin is a hormone created by the pancreas which regulates glucose (sugar) levels in our bloodstream. Though once believed to be an obsolete component of milk production, research in recent years has shown that it is, in fact, a contributing hormone in the production of breastmilk. As your body begins to produce milk, glans in the breast become highly sensitive to insulin levels in the body. Thus, moms who are dealing with diabetes or are pre-diabetic are more likely to experience supply difficulties (even if nursing frequently) and experience an overall delay in milk production. Fluctuating glucose levels in moms can make it harder for a substantial supply for their newborns — thus, initiating the use of supplemental entities (such as formula or breastfeeding banks) as the milk slowly comes in. Fortunately, taking insulin while nursing is safe for both mom and baby and helps to ensure that moms are able to achieve their nursing goals.

Cortisol is a hormone released when the brain experiences stress and in response to low blood-glucose concentration. Though stress itself cannot be passed on to our babies via breastmilk, components of the hormone are said to pass from mom to infant during nursing. Thus, breastfed babies are found to have higher levels of the hormone than formula fed babies. What's most important to take away from the cortisol hormone is not that it negatively impacts baby (as breastmilk will always be the more preferred option in optimum feeding choices when possible) — but the more stressed and the higher the cortisol levels, the more impact it will have on milk production. Though stress is inherent in motherhood, the more we find ways in which to mitigate things outside of our control (i.e. via meditation, nursing in a quiet space, listening to relaxing music, taking a walk, et cetera), the less likely our stress levels will negatively impact milk production and supply.

Oxytocin, aka the love hormone, plays a huge role in the breastfeeding experience. During labor and delivery, oxytocin levels surge to initiate contractions, to relieve the body of the pain associated with those very contractions and aids in strengthening the uterus to help push baby out (as noted in detail in the *Oxytocin and The Power of the Mind* chapter of *Hello, Hello: The Inspirational Guide to Delivery*). Immediately after delivery, oxytocin levels rise to an unmatchable level—

oftentimes sending moms into a state of euphoria that can only be reached in childbirth.

When nursing, oxytocin is what encourages contractions of the breast glans that secrete breast milk. As baby begins to nurse, nerves in your breast send a signal to your brain to release the hormone. Oxytocin sends a signal to your breast glans to begin contracting — leading to the **let-down** (the sensation moms feel as their milk begins to reach and push through the nipples). The longer you nurse, the more oxytocin released in your body. The increase in this love hormone tends to cause moms to feel relaxed and/or sleepy when breastfeeding and also raises your body temperature (hence, why many of us sweat while we nurse).

This increase in body temperature also tends to make moms thirsty while nursing — again stressing the importance of staying hydrated as your milk supply regulates. Even when you aren't nursing, oxytocin can cause you to let-down even if baby isn't present. The sound of their cry, looking at a picture, or simply thinking about something they did that day can contribute to an unplanned let-down (*Note: It's great to invest in nipple pads to keep you dry in case you start to leak, but remember to change them often as to prevent moisture buildup, which can lead to thrush or clogged milk ducts.*) If you start to leak and you don't have any nipple pads, simply push on your nipple until the let down as stopped.

Colostrum

The initial milk your body will produce during the first few days post-delivery is **colostrum**. If you were to pump, you would notice this milk is more yellow in color. Hello, Hello liquid gold! Colostrum is magical — another reminder of just how incredible your body is. Your colostrum is filled with tons of antibodies that:

> A. protects your newborn from bacteria and viruses as they enter the world (especially important for babies born in hospitals)
>
> B. has a laxative effect to help your newborn expel **meconium** (their first poop that looks like tar, which could take up to three days to fully pass)

Many moms and for good reason, refer to colostrum as their baby's first vaccine. Your baby will drink colostrum for the first 3-4 days until your mature milk starts to come in (cue: engorgement). Though it will be low in volume, it's full of vitamins baby will need.

Early Struggles

Whether you're planning to breastfeed or not, your body will begin the milk production process. Many women fear they aren't producing enough milk. This is usually unlikely if baby is eating. If you're experiencing latching issues with your newborn, consulting a lactation specialist or your midwife and / or doula will be of great help. Taking a nursing class (there are many online as well) prior to baby being born can be of the utmost help in preparation for feeding and latching positions. There are times when the milk supply is low and this is often made evident by a newborn not gaining enough weight or becoming frustrated during nursing sessions (likely not getting full enough). Wherever you fall in the spectrum, it's imperative not to stress.

There are varied reasons whereby your milk supply may be delayed. Yet, a delay in production does not equate to failure of breastfeeding. The more you continue to attempt to nurse, the more your body will produce milk. The less you try, the more you supplement and the more stressed you become about your supply, the less you'll produce. Though it reads very straight forward, it can be daunting trying to understand why your production is slower than others.

The level of stress mothers experience during this time is understandable (we all just want the best start for our babies), but it's also the very thing that stalls milk production. The less you stress and realize the process is normal and the more you try to simply take it day by day with continuous feeding, the process will start. Try not to be overwhelmed by doctors, family or friends — baby will get what they need. Just keep going. Relax and breathe.

While the stress of day to day can gravely impact milk production delays, certain medical conditions can be the cause as well. These may include:

- **High levels of stress caused by traumatic birthing experiences.** Unfortunately, traumatic birthing experiences are all too common in an age where medical advances are at their peak. The fact that the birthing process is treated as a severe medical condition often leads to unnecessary steps in interventions. This has the potential to cause horrid experiences including unplanned cesarean sections, the use of unwanted tools during the pushing stage, or extremely long and painful labors. The increase of stress hormones released in the body during delivery can lead to a drop in hormones needed to produce milk; thus, delaying milk production.

- **Retained fragments of the placenta.** Post-delivery of our placenta, doctors and midwives first order of business is to ensure the entire placenta has been delivered or surgically removed. Any bits retained in the uterus could lead to life threatening internal hemorrhage. If parts of the placenta remain attached to the uterus, the body will not release the sudden drop of progesterone which initiates milk production. This is an extreme instance whereby milk production is stalled. Fortunately, it doesn't happen often as placentas are examined thoroughly post-delivery.

- **High levels of pain medication, IV fluids, or hemorrhage.** Fluid levels in our bodies can impact milk production as well. If a mother experienced high levels of blood loss, it may impact the body's ability to release proper hormones to trigger lactation. If a mother has been given high levels of medication and/or high levels of intravenous fluids, it will take longer for the body to rid of the fluids prior to allowing for the release of milk production and let-down.

- **Premature delivery.** If you delivered baby prematurely, it's still likely your milk will come in, but it may delay milk production if your body hasn't started producing colostrum — depending on how early the baby was born. If your milk has come in, you may only be able to nurse via pumping, which can make it harder to produce a substantial milk supply. Though it may be much harder, it's still possible.

- **Delays in seeing your baby.** There are times when a mother cannot be with her baby within the first hours or days post-delivery. If you're unable to nurse immediately, pumping or using your hands to literally push/express the milk out of your breasts will help to encourage milk production. The longer a mother goes without expressing (or releasing) the milk from the breasts, the stronger the signal the body receives that it doesn't need to produce any. This is often referred to as *supply and demand.* The body supplies what is demanded of it.

- **Previous breast surgery or procedure.** Moms who have had breast augmentation surgeries or medical occurrences that led to breast surgery, may have issues with scar tissue or blocked ducts from past procedures. The good news is that if you have had surgery in the past, it's still possible to nurse — though it may be harder. I had a tumor removed from my left breast at 16 years old. I was able to nurse both of my babies, but the scar tissue made it much harder to express and pump. The start of my nursing journey wasn't a walk in the park, but it was in that moment where I felt like I couldn't go on, that I was able to push through. It may be harder, but it's not impossible.

If you are someone who has experienced any of the situations aforementioned, the great news is that with help, patience and support, you still have the possibility of nursing baby if that is your goal. For those who have not experienced the cases mentioned, this may signify you need to express more milk in order for your body to produce more. The goal is to try and relax as much as humanly possible a which can be extremely hard to do. If you strive to just let it be, it can take huge amounts of pressure off of you as a new mom. Whether you're being hounded to breastfeed or not, you must surround yourself with a strong support system that will encourage whatever dreams you have about this experience.

In the end, you should never give up your dream to nurse and should always follow your heart. Speak with other moms who have struggled with nursing (most moms) and you'll learn that sometimes you just have to push through the pain and the struggle. For many women who were able to make it past the hard start, the moment they felt like they couldn't take the pain any longer was when it became easier. Nursing is a journey and it's an ever-evolving one.

An easy start may have many bumps in the road, whereas a hard beginning could result in smooth sailing soon thereafter. Try not to judge your start and don't beat yourself up if it doesn't happen the way you planned. Just have faith and empowered thoughts. Know that it may be hard, but this is your fight and you'll overcome. Breastfeeding is just the start of the many sacrifices you'll make as a mom to ensure the best result for baby. You got this!

Engorgement, Cabbage, and Clogged Milk Ducts

Now that the colostrum phase has passed (typically 3-4 days, sometimes longer), your body will start to produce mature milk. **Engorgement** is normally the first sign of this transition, as your breasts fill up an unusual and uncomfortable amount. During this time, your breasts get overfull (of milk, blood and fluids), become huge, hard and painful. At the end of the day, it sucks. Thankfully, this is a great sign that your body is doing what it's supposed to do — and it's only temporary.

Express and feed is the focus, as it will aid in softening the breasts during engorgement. Though you can become engorged at any point during your breastfeeding journey (i.e. missing a session once baby starts to sleep through the night), nothing quite feels like the initial phase. Fortunately, one of the greatest assets you can have during this time is **cabbage**. Cabbage is an herbal, holistic method to aid in engorgement with its anti-inflammatory properties that will help to reduce the swelling, pain and reduce your milk supply (hence, the importance of only using the cabbage during your engorged days or when trying to reduce an oversupply of milk). Have someone buy cabbage from the store, place in the refrigerator and when cold, apply the cabbage leaves directly to your breasts several times a day. Ice packs and anti-inflammatory pain medication may also help to alleviate pain as well. Remember to ensure that your medication of choice is applicable to your nursing.

It's important to remember that, as you're engorged, **you must get the milk out of your breasts**. Removing your milk (via nursing, pumping, or hand expression) will aid in easing the discomfort and help to avoid painful **clogged milk ducts**. Maintaining proper release/flow of your milk is similar to avoiding a car jam. If you wait too long to nurse or pump, or if you don't expel enough milk, you can develop a blockage of milk flow in a duct that prevents it from reaching the nipple. This backed up milk duct is tender and painful and can be sucked out by baby or massaged out when pumping or nursing.

If you develop clogged ducts at any time during your breastfeeding experience, you must continue to nurse even amidst the pain; for the longer it remains clogged, the higher your chances of developing an infection. Using ice on a clogged duct (placing it on your nipple) to numb the area or physically pinching the clogged duct right before nursing can help mitigate some of the pain that occurs during the initial latch. Warm compresses, warm showers and massages are beneficial in removing the duct, which can be identified by a small lump in the breast. One of the best ways to relieve a clog is to lay baby on their back and nurse on all fours (allowing gravity and baby's sucking to help pull the clog out). Once the clog is out, the pain usually subsides; but the healing process varies for everyone. With my very first clogged duct, the moment it was released, the pain immediately subsided. With my second clogged duct, once it was released, my nipple was sore (feeling extremely bruised) for about two weeks. Again, it's different for everyone and even every clog.

The goal is never to get too backed up — which is easier said than done. Sometimes having help at the house can backfire in terms of milk production and flow. If someone is staying the night to help, you may get a full night's sleep while the baby is bottle fed during their nighttime feeding. This could possibly impact your milk production (if done over a long period of time) and cause clogged milk ducts (if you aren't pumping throughout the night). Severely clogged milk ducts could lead to a painful infection of the breasts called **mastitis,** which can also be caused by bacteria entering the breast (i.e. bacteria from baby's mouth entering through a crack on the nipple).

Ensuring that baby is eating enough, latched on and sucking correctly, maintaining the constant removal of milk from your breasts and making sure to allow enough time on each breast during your nursing sessions can help to avoid infection caused by a clogged duct.

Continuing to nurse or express your milk frequently can help to minimize the pain of engorgement in the first few days of your mature milk coming in and throughout your nursing journey. Hand expression (taking your hands and pushing the milk from the top of your breasts down and out of the nipple) can help to relieve the pressure as well — seeing as though many moms struggle with pumping during the initial phase of engorgement. Whatever you do, don't skip a nursing session. If baby is sleeping and you have the energy, pump or hand express into a bottle or breastmilk freezer bag and place it in your freezer for later use. You can never have too much breastmilk in the beginning: just save and freeze! Your milk can last in the freezer up to 9 months—which can be a huge help if you're going back to work while continuing to breastfeed.

Be Fearless: Tips to Help You

Whatever thoughts you have going into your breastfeeding journey will certainly come to pass. If you're fearful and have negative thoughts going into the process, it will likely pan out that way. If you go into the journey feeling empowered, you'll have that very experience. This doesn't mean it will be easy or stress free. But it will set up the foundation by which your experience is built — ensuring you can and will overcome the hurdles that will arise. The following is a list I've developed to help empower your thoughts before or during your journey; things to help you find your light at the end of the tunnel:

Yes, it will be hard and sometimes painful.

The beginning of the journey is always an interesting one. As with anything new, there is a trial and error phase, whereby you and baby will have to figure out your flow. Once you both find your rhythm, things will get easier. In the beginning, you probably will only feed baby in a certain position(s) on the bed, in a chair, with a certain breastfeeding pillow or boppy, et cetera. You'll probably see other moms who are doing all kinds of things while breastfeeding (walking around, doing laundry, hosting a dinner party, et cetera) and wonder how on earth they make it look so easy.

The great news is that, over time, your nipples won't be as tender and you'll be able to do more simultaneously. Don't rush the process and don't ever compare your journey. It will get better if you can just push through your hardest moments. Don't give up. You are not alone and there are countless mothers who have either already experienced what you have, or are going through the same things concurrently. Reach out for help and avoid keeping your struggles internal. Sharing your feelings may help you discover the trick to turn your whole world upside down in the best way. And if you feel like you need to stop, then stop. Don't put pressure on yourself to do something to appease anyone else's opinions on your journey. This is about you and your baby.

This is YOUR body. Honor it.

From day one, freeze your milk.

Your body makes milk based on supply and demand. However, much baby eats (demands), is how much your body will produce (supplies). It's truly an incredible process (hence, how mothers of multiples can produce enough milk for their babies). Typically, within the first four months or so, you may have an oversupply of milk as your body figures out how much to produce to sufficiently feed baby. In order to have a supply, your body pulls all of the nutrients it needs (including calcium from your bones) to produce your milk. Simply put, it's exhausting. Pumping coupled with nursing is extremely exhausting and there tends to be a lot of pressure to start to build the milk bunker once it's time to go back to work or simply enjoy some free time.

A trick to help build your milk bunker in the freezer without feeling completely overwhelmed by last minute pumping, or over doing it in the early days: *set a goal for just one bottle a day* (doesn't matter how many ounces). If you, like most women, have excess milk in the morning, before or after nursing, hand express or pump some milk into a bottle. Use that same bottle throughout the day if you ever feel the urge to express or pump more milk. If all you get is the milk from the morning, great! At the end of each day, pour the milk you pumped into a milk freezer bag, date and store. Eventually, you'll fall into a rhythm and soon discover that you have months' worth of milk. *NOTE: Small amounts of milk can come in handy when baby has a cold by adding to their food, or shooting the milk up their nose!*

Establishing a more realistic and less stringent way to freeze milk will also come in handy when your body regulates its milk production. Needing to freeze milk with an oversupply will always come in handy (whether it's for rainy days, to use when making their food, or even to donate to other moms who may be struggling with their supply). Trying to freeze milk after your supply has regulated can be extremely hard and severely stressful (and the more stressed the harder to produce milk). If you find a rhythm of pumping once a day during the early months, your milk supply will likely regulate itself to match that demand as well. Around the 4-6 month mark postpartum, prolactin levels in most moms start to decrease to help regulate supply. As many moms go back to work around six months, already having a full bunker can alleviate tons of stress and can even be helpful in transitioning baby from breast to bottle or sippy cup.

NOTE: Prolactin levels are higher than normal during breastfeeding which stalls ovulation, reduces progesterone levels and stores extra fat for milk production. Higher levels of prolactin often result in a lower metabolism (resulting in weight gain or extreme struggles for weight loss), even though the act of nursing helps moms burn upwards of 500 calories a day. High cortisol levels (stress) also increases prolactin levels, sometimes making it harder to lose weight. Every journey is different — some will have the weight melt away during nursing while others don't. Try not to compare your body to anyone else's. You're doing incredible work for baby. Over time, your body will start to regulate its hormone levels. More on weight gain and loss soon.

A major goal in sustaining a healthy supply is to avoid becoming overwhelmed by the prospect of producing milk. The more stressed, the less milk you can produce. Freezing your milk can help bring about a lot of relief and doing it in a manageable way can help reduce your stress levels. If you can't nurse and pump, that's okay! Your baby is still receiving what they need. Even if your nursing stint is short, that too is okay! Babies who are formula fed are able to survive and thrive the same as breastfed babies. Though there are inherent benefits to the natural properties of breastmilk which is tailor made for your baby, there are also benefits to women who chose to end nursing early or chose formula overall. Follow your heart, listen to your gut and don't feel bullied into doing anything that you know doesn't work with you and baby's needs.

Feed on demand (and wherever you need to).

There are many methods parents use to get their baby on a schedule. I'm a strong believer parents should do whatever helps establish as much order and sanity as humanly possible. Allowing you baby to nurse whenever they're hungry will help to establish a strong milk supply. Allowing babies to feed on demand also helps to establish a routine through time as they get older and find a rhythm. It's always best never to feel pressured into anyone else's method for feeding. If you decide to feed on a strict schedule, be sure to hand express or pump frequently as not to minimize your milk production. If feeding on demand becomes too overwhelming (i.e. if baby can grub!), then allow some of those feedings to be with a bottle. While someone else is feeding your baby with the bottle, hand express, pump, or just rest. All in all, remember to avoid allowing your breasts to become too full, which could lead to clogged ducts or mastitis.

It's also essential to feed baby wherever you are. If baby is hungry and you have the capacity to physically feed them, then do so. Period. As people start to evolve in their thinking towards motherhood and as more women become stronger in their resolve to feed their babies when and where they need, it will continue to become less of a dramatic occasion. Most times, people won't notice. It's hard to decipher whether a mom is feeding or simply holding her baby. If you feel more comfortable with a cover, then use one. If baby gets too hot being so covered up, then find other ways to make yourself and baby comfortable (whatever that entails). People's lack of understanding, concern, or simple kindness should never prevent you from doing what you need to do for baby. Handle your business.

Keep your nipples dry, post feeding (tips to prevent cracking or infection).

Cracked and sore nipples can be extremely discouraging during your breastfeeding journey. Fortunately, a few tips can help to alleviate the pain and help to avoid damage:

- Prior to nursing and pumping (more so in the first few months as your nipples adjust), **use a natural form of lubrication** (i.e. organic nipple creams that are safe for babies). By keeping your nipples lightly moisturized prior to feeding or pumping, it can help to prevent cracking—which occurs when your baby or the pump is constantly tugging on dry nipples.

- Post feedings, **before putting your bra back on, wipe your nipples dry or allow them to air dry.** Placing your bra on top of moist nipples can lead to infection — such as **thrush** (a yeast like infection caused by overgrown fungus on the nipple). This can lead to painful, sharp sensations in the breast and can also cause baby to develop thrush as well.

  ‣ *NOTE: Breastfed babies are more likely to develop thrush, as it passes back and forth between mom and baby during nursing.*

  ‣ Wiping the inside of baby's mouth with a dry burp cloth post feedings can help to avoid thrush. Natural remedies, like grapefruit seed extract, can be just as or more beneficial in ridding of the infection versus prescribed medication.

> ‣ Many moms and babies develop thrush at some point, so don't stress. With a little research and patience, you'll find what works best for you both.

- If your nipples are extremely sore for a long period of time, it may be an indicator that you should **<u>try a different nursing position with baby</u>** — as they may not be latching correctly. Connecting with a lactation specialist, your midwife, doula or other moms can help to discover the issues you and baby may be facing when it comes to latching. Sometimes underlying issues such as a short frenulum in baby's mouth may be the culprit.

A short frenulum may be the cause for some discomfort.

During the first few pediatric visits, the doctor will check baby's **frenulum** (the tissue which is found under the top lip and under the tongue). If it's too short, your pediatrician may suggest getting it clipped. If so, baby will visit a specialist who will perform the clipping in a procedure that lasts no more than three minutes—whereby you can immediately place baby back on your breast to nurse. This will calm the baby and help illustrate if the shortened frenulum was to blame for the latching struggles.

Pay attention to your breasts, and treat them care.

Milk blisters (small bumps on or around the nipple) can be extremely painful. It's a sign that you have clogged milk duct, which will have to be released.

<u>**Try the ice method**</u>: place ice on the area for numbing and then squeeze your nipple as your baby latches. Try to get your nipple far inside of their mouth to ensure good latching and to help prevent them from biting your nipple. Also, try <u>nursing on all fours</u> with baby on their back, to allow gravity to aid in baby sucking out the clog.

If you have severe cracking (and/or bleeding), <u>**only wash your nipples with soap and water**</u>. Don't use lotions (only baby friendly nipple creams prior to nursing). You want to try and allow the area to heal as much as possible, so it may be best to hand express during this time—while baby drinks your milk from a bottle. This can be helpful in transitioning baby to be able to drink from both the breast and bottle (especially useful when you have to be away for any amount of time).

Though many may advise against giving babies both breast and bottle early on (referring to nipple confusion), babies adjust quickly and very well — and are extremely smart. Their adaptability helps them to make the proper connection for both. The earlier you get baby on breast and bottle, the easier it will be for them to use the bottle whenever it's necessary (giving you some free time — and preventing them from being completely dependent on your breasts for feeding). Remember to hand express often to keep your milk production strong. Pumping can cause damage to the nipples as well (especially if you pump for too long or they're extremely dry). Hand expression is a great tool. *NOTE: Moisturize your breasts prior to hand expression as not to make your skin too dry.*

If you have inverted nipples, it doesn't mean you can never breastfeed. It may make the process a bit harder and you may have to come up with creative ways to get your nipples in the best latching position. But with time, persistence and help from others with the same experience, you can find what works best for you and have an incredibly empowering experience!

Stay hydrated and eat well.

One of the most important things to remember during this time is that your body will do whatever it needs to produce milk. Your body will draw calcium from your bones if it has to in order to produce milk for baby. Back in the day, women's diets were so low in calcium that they would lose their teeth due to their body extracting so much calcium from their bones. This clearly doesn't happen anymore, but rather stresses the importance of eating a well-balanced diet, rich in calcium. Introducing a calcium magnesium vitamin can help to fill the void in your diet, as well as helping to stimulate a healthy digestive tract — more information on this in the *Vitamins (+ Healthy Eating)* chapter.

It's essential to provide your body with what it needs in order not to become completely depleted of nutrients. **Dieting** will cause your body to store even more fat in order to ensure it can produce milk — hence, why dieting during nursing can cause you to actually gain weight. Adding extra healthy calories can help to alleviate becoming overly tired and drained from the process. With your body doing so much work producing milk, to the physical act of nursing, it adds an extra level of exhaustion. With so much going on, one of the areas you should try not to stress about is your weight (especially within the first couple of months postpartum). Soon enough, you'll have time to solely focus on losing all of the weight. Remember this is just a season. Focus on the importance of health and nourishment for breastfeeding. And when the time comes, you can eat according to your personal goals and desires.

It's also essential to stay hydrated during your nursing journey — especially in the beginning as your body adjust to the extreme hormonal changes. Reducing caffeine intakes and increasing your healthy fluid intake (i.e. water, electrolytes, et cetera) will help to ensure your body replenishes all of the nourishment it releases during milk production. During the early days of breastfeeding, you'll feel extremely dehydrated while your nurse. You may also experience hot flashes and sweat often, especially during let-down. Remember to ALWAYS have a bottle of water with you when you nurse during the first couple of months. You'll feel extremely thirsty during your nursing sessions due to your higher levels of prolactin and staying hydrated will help to reduce the likelihood of a drop in your milk supply.

NOTE: Remember to empty your bladder prior to nursing to help avoid your bladder becoming too full — especially when drinking water during your nursing session.

Find ways to encourage your let-down.

Sometimes one of the hardest parts of nursing — especially when you need to hand express or pump, or when you have a really fussy baby who is upset that the milk isn't coming out fast enough — is the let-down. In the first weeks and months of nursing, many moms experience the sensation of the milk pushing down toward the nipple in preparation for feeding. While some moms don't have a specific feeling during let-down, others may experience a tingling or burning sensation in the nipple area, cramping (due to uterine contractions), extreme thirst, or a noticeable difference in the manner by which baby is sucking (slowing down with noticeable and audible gulps).

There are times, especially during engorgement, when encouraging the let-down is hard — thus, making it harder to express your milk. A few tips that may aid in fostering your let down include:

 ▸ **Take a deep breath right before you nurse.** The more you can relax, the easier your let-down can flow. Conversely, the more you stress, the harder it will be (which may also impact your overall milk production).

 ▸ **Place a warm compress on your breasts** to encourage milk flow. A warm shower is also helpful in generating your let-down.

 ▸ **Smell your baby** - yup it could work. The sensation of smelling, hearing, or even looking at baby can encourage your let-down.

‣ **<u>Finding a less distracting place to nurse</u>**, that keeps you calm and anxiety-free, will significantly aid in your let-down.

‣ **<u>Massage your breasts prior to nursing</u>.**

Pay attention to your baby's reaction to your milk.

Take note of how baby responds to your milk. If baby responds adversely during a particular nursing session, it could signify a food sensitivity to something you ate previously. Typically, if a food makes you gassy, it will likely make baby gassy as well. Avoiding gassy foods such as cabbage, broccoli, or brussel sprouts, can help to alleviate gas pains in your baby.

If baby has a sensitive tummy, experiences intense colic, or has painful acid reflux and throws up an abnormal amount, it may help to simply adjust your eating habits for a while. An idea of what to avoid in order to simplify your diet to accommodate a sensitive baby includes (but is not limited to):

‣ dairy

‣ onion

‣ garlic

‣ gassy green vegetables

‣ sugar (processed foods)

‣ acidic foods (ie: oranges or tomatoes)

Following a regiment similar to that listed above can be a great source, especially during the first few months when babies experience colic. **Colic** is severe pain and discomfort caused by gas in the tummy or digestive tract issues. Many babies are colicky within the first month or so. If baby suddenly has crying spells that last for hours at a time (seemingly for no reason at all), try not to get discouraged. Colic is trying for your newborn, just as much as it can be for your sanity.

Though it may seem like you can't take the crying anymore, it's important to do whatever you need in order to find patience and calmness. If that means going outside alone for some fresh air, handing baby to a spouse or family member, or just closing your eyes and taking in deep breaths, you must find patience and mind your energy. Your baby will feed off of the energy you put forth — so, the calmer you are, the calmer they will get. If you have anxiety, they will feel it. Fortunately, there are some methods to help with colic in your newborn (along with your adjusted eating habits). These include but are not limited to:

- Adding a tummy massage and leg compressions to your daily routine (whether in the mornings or at night). This can help to get the gas moving in the intestinal tract. A quick search online can offer you a vast array of techniques for baby's massage. If the uncomfortably lasts beyond the colicky phase, Craniosacral therapy (typically around four months) may be beneficial for your little one.

- Homeopathic remedies may be helpful as well (i.e. gripe waters, or non-habit forming remedies for acid reflux).

- Holding babies in specialty positions can aid in pain relief as well. For example, hold baby with their back to your belly. Pull their legs upward so they're in a seated position in your arms. Using your free hand, add some pressure to their belly area. They will release a lot of gas as the pressure helps to get things moving in their intestinal tract. Or, allowing baby to lay, tummy down, on your knees or forearms can help to relieve gas pressure. A quick search online can offer more techniques on alleviating newborn gas.

Remember how blessed you are to have this experience.

Breastfeeding is not an easy feat. Your body is producing an exact match for baby's needs — even changing its properties when you or baby gets sick to ensure a stronger immune system. Even in knowing how special this moment is, it can still become extremely frustrating and isolating. Intense feelings and thoughts can pop up in your mind during this time and it's important to be honest with your emotions and mental state. During the hardest moments, it's imperative to remember just how blessed we are for this experience. There are many moms who physically aren't capable of nursing — those who aren't able to commit to breastfeeding due to work schedules or a lack of support — and even those who have to deal with a milk supply after losing a baby.

In any case, it's essential to keep an empowered perspective. Remembering that there are countless women who would give anything to have this experience may help to strengthen your resolve when you can't see the light at the end of the tunnel. It may not be easy, but we are so fortunate to have this moment.

All in all, breastfeeding is work!

How you feel is appropriate, valid and normal. Thoughts you have in those dark moments have probably been expressed by more women then you know. It's not about being perfectly joyful at all times — that's not realistic nor necessary. It's simply about what you do with those thoughts and how you constantly work to train and retrain your habitual thinking. For what we constantly think, is who we become. And it's important to strive to become our truest, most empowered selves for the sake of ourselves and our baby.

Remember that every phase of motherhood is a season. And once you overcome one season, there is another right around the corner to tackle. It's a never-ending journey. So remind yourself of how special this time is, because it will be over soon. Honor this time and honor yourself. Take your time, trust your power and allow your vulnerability to become your greatest motivation. Your baby and your body will thank you later. You got this! I promise you do.

Focus on the benefits.

There are often times when the benefits to nursing your little one outweigh the adversity. As you know, your body will produce milk that is specific to the needs of your baby (their best source of immunity). There are also times when it's hard to find reasons to continue on.

Aside from being a perfect match to your baby, there are other quantifiable benefits to nursing — even when it seems daunting:

- breastmilk is rich in antibodies that help protect baby against disease
- includes proteins for baby's physical and developmental growth
- houses carbs, fats and minerals for their brain and nervous system development
- aids in increased protection for baby from:
  - allergies
  - bacterial meningitis
  - Chrons disease
  - increased cases of diaper rash
  - diarrhea and constipation (though both can occur in a breastfed baby if they are reacting to something in your diet or fighting off a virus)
  - ear infection
  - eczema
  - juvenile diabetes
  - respiratory infection
  - SIDS
  - urinary tract infections

There are also extraordinary benefits for you as well, including but not limited to:

- encouraging uterine contractions post-delivery — which is imperative to preventing hemorrhage

- helping some moms lose more of the baby weight faster (seeing as though your body burns extra calories during each nursing session) — remember that each body is different and responds uniquely to nursing

- oxytocin released during breastfeeding helps to shrink the uterus back to its pre-pregnancy shape sooner

- nursing aids in delayed ovulation — meaning no periods for a while (upwards of 9 months); but please keep in mind **you absolutely can get pregnant while breastfeeding**

- helps to increase bonding between mom and baby as this special moment in time can only happen with you (you possess the magical powers to sooth baby at any given second — it's extremely special)

- recent studies continue to show that breastfeeding lowers the chances of developing breast cancer

Formula (another great option)

With all of the benefits that both you and baby receive from nursing, it's understandable why so many moms stress themselves into a frenzy about the breastfeeding journey. No single journey is the same, but many are alike. If you're someone who physically cannot or chooses not to breastfeed, it doesn't make you any less of a mom. What is most important to take away is that, you can only best parent when you're the closest to your best self holistically (physically, mentally, emotionally and spiritually). This plays out differently for every single mom — depending on your birthing experience, health history, emotional and mental stability, personal needs, support system, et cetera.

What is important is that baby is fed. If you must do formula, then do formula! Though there are more immediate benefits to breastmilk, formula is the difference between life and death for some. I personally was a formula fed baby, who breastfed both of my babies. But if it weren't for formula, my mother would not have had a way to feed me due to severe health complications she was facing at the time. Though it may not have been ideal, she did what she had to do as a mother in order for me to live and thrive.

Not having been breastfed is not something that I remember nor hold over my mother's head. The same goes for baby. They won't remember it and they won't hate you for it. Do what you need to do to ensure the best start and strongest foundation and never allow yourself to feel ashamed. There are setbacks to both nursing and using formula and each scenario has obstacles to overcome. Find what works best of you and baby and do just that. Fortunately, these days there are stronger options for formulas that are less harsh on a baby's maturing gut. While most formulas cause constipation in babies, organic, holistic options may not. Also, doing research into donation centers that offer unused breastmilk from other moms may be a viable option as well.

With judgment of moms choosing formula, there also tends to be a judgment centered around how long we choose to nurse as well. Don't ever feel like you have to defend your choice to nurse, use formula, or to do both. Breastfeed for however long YOU decide. If someone has anything to say about how long or short you breastfeed with a judgmental eye, they shouldn't be in your support system anyway. No one else matters in this equation. This is your body and you must listen to it throughout the entire journey. Whether it's a three month, six month or 36 month journey, it is yours and baby's. And at the end of the day it's simply up to you. You are superwoman and the only kryptonite you have is in your mind. Mind your thoughts and strengthen your spirit. You got this!

Exclusive Pumping

One particular area in regards to nourishing our babies that often goes overlooked, is **exclusive pumping** (solely pumping rather than breastfeeding). There are many reasons whereby moms choose to exclusively pump their breastmilk. This is often a necessity for mothers of premature babies or those in newborn intensive care units (NICU) recovering and those with consistent latching complications. Whatever the reason, it's always a personal one — and a strong one at that. Exclusively pumping is a hard feat to tackle and moms who choose this route have to overcome many physical and psychological battles to have an empowered experience.

Exclusive pumping includes having to regulate and manage your own milk supply void of the natural properties that occur when nursing. This happens via pumping upwards of 12 times a day in the early months. Essentially, when a mom isn't burping, changing diapers, putting baby down for a nap, or any of the other tasks involved with newborns, she is pretty much glued to her pump. This can take a huge mental toll on someone, no matter how special the moment is. It's physically taxing and mentally draining, as you have to develop a love and normalcy about your new and very demanding routine.

The hardships of pumping include having to constantly monitor your milk production (which is typically only noticeable if a baby is losing weight when breastfeeding — since you can never truly tell how many ounces they're getting). Other struggles include having to find a rhythm that doesn't negatively impact milk supply, pumping throughout the night, cleaning the pump and parts daily (which is way more exhausting then it sounds) and having to keep track of the feeding schedule versus the pumping schedule. It's hard and it's essential to allow yourself the opportunity to find what works best for you in a loving and compassionate way. Exclusive pumping is not the easy way out. It's an extremely selfless and exhausting feat and you should be proud of yourself for accomplishing however long the journey lasts.

The great thing about exclusive pumping is that it gets easier with time. As with every aspect of motherhood, the more you repeat something, the more engrained it'll become into your psyche and routine. If you're able to make it through the first few weeks of exclusive pumping, chances are you're going to be able to continue until you're ready to stop. Whenever that is and for whatever reason that may be, you must listen to your body, mind your well-being and care for your holistic self. When the time comes, go with it and never be ashamed.

As with anything, there are benefits to exclusive pumping. For example, by exclusively breastfeeding, there are times when you may not have the ease or flexibility to leave baby with a spouse, parent, friend, et cetera, in order to enjoy some time for yourself — especially if baby uses you as a pacifier. Exclusively pumping depends on the bottle — thus, you won't always have to physically be present in order for baby to eat.

Finding other moms who have chosen this path and speaking with lactation specialists on how to best serve yourself, treat and care for your nipples and finding and/or maintaining some sort of emotional and psychological stability can be a grave help in pushing through your journey. The fact that one would choose such a hard feat is something that should never be taken lightly. It's completely commendable for mothers to do this and it's imperative you commend yourself should you become one in this community as well. It's also important to remember that starting your journey exclusively pumping doesn't ensure that it will end that way. Continuously trying to find a means to nurse and pump can be a realistic goal. But whatever the goal, just know that you can do it!

How to Increase Milk Supply

One of the most stressful components of breastfeeding is your milk supply: having too much or not enough. It's scary to think you may not have enough and it can be overwhelming to have too much. Either way, it can always seem as though the grass is greener on the other side of the spectrum. The truth is that both can be stressful and hard to deal with.

The following offers some remedies to aid in **increasing your milk supply**:

Reduce stress.

The more stressed you find yourself, the more your milk supply will take a hit (taking into account the normal stress levels associated with newborns). <u>The more you stress about not producing enough, the harder it will be to start producing more.</u> If the moment arises where you feel completely overwhelmed about your supply, take a deep breath and remember: it's not the end of the world. Your journey may not go exactly as planned and there may be times where sticking it out doesn't offer enough nourishment to baby. In those times it may seem like your world is crashing if you have to supplement. Yet, no matter how bad you want to exclusively breastfeed, having to supplement (and having the capability of doing so) is just as powerful. Never minimize the fullness of the work you do to ensure the strongest start for baby. Try the tips below and allow nature to take its course (wherever that course leads you). Your journey is unique and it may deviate from your initial plans. Allow your anticipations to evolve and give yourself space to adjust and adapt according to your circumstances.

Nurse more frequently and offer both sides.

As you now expertly know, your milk production is about supply and demand. Increasing your nursing sessions (and possibly the length of time on each breast) can help to increase your body's need to produce more milk. And remember to offer both breasts during each session.

Ensure baby has a good latch.

The key to successful nursing is a successful latch. This ensures that the milk is actually flowing, which will aid in increased milk production. Finding lactation specialists, help groups and other moms can be vital for you and baby's success.

Take a "nursing vacation".

For a few days straight, you'll relax in your bed (or wherever is most comfortable) and nurse as frequently as you can. Essentially, that is your primary focus: to nurse and/or pump. Typically, around day two or three you'll notice an increase in your supply. Remember to stay hydrated and eat well during this time.

Replace the pacifier with your nipple.

When baby would normally need a pacifier for soothing, replace it with your nipple. The suction sensation from baby will encourage your body to produce more milk.

Only offer your breasts.

Don't offer a bottle during any of your nursing sessions. Your baby needs to nurse with you, as they can get more milk via nursing than hand expression or pumping.

Stay hydrated and mind your eating.

Your health is imperative for milk production. There is no need to overly-hydrate, but it's essential to avoid becoming dehydrated or not eating enough. The more nutrients your body has to pull from, the less taxing it will be on you physically. The more iron rich foods you add to your diet, the more likely you are to increase your milk supply. You're capable of working on your weight-loss goals while nursing, but it's essential to avoid depriving your body of what it needs to successfully produce your supply (i.e. extreme dieting).

Express/pump before or after your nursing session.

You don't need a physical pump in order to effectively remove milk from your breasts. Hand expression is just as powerful of a tool and can allow you to manipulate the milk from your breast in better ways. Many experts suggest expressing or pumping milk post nursing sessions. If that is too hard, try before the nursing session.

NOTE: You may hear a lot about your **foremilk** and **hindmilk**. That is simply referring to milk in the beginning of your feeding session versus milk at the end. The longer the feed, the higher the fat content (hindmilk), leaving them more satisfied for longer periods of time. Choosing to hand express or pump before or after your nursing session is completely up to you. Either way will aid in increasing your milk supply, and both the foremilk and hindmilk will be extremely beneficial to your baby. Remember to store and freeze the extra milk you pump as well!

Add oatmeal to your diet.

Oatmeal is not only an easy choice for breakfast, but adding it to your diet can help to increase milk supply. There are also many food/snack choices you can find in baby stores or online that focus on increasing milk supply. For example, when nursing my first born, my milk supply took a dip when he started to sleep throughout the night. So, I made homemade lactation cookies. Essentially, the combination of oats, Brewer's yeast and flaxseed were key to increasing my supply. Remember that every journey is different. If the oatmeal doesn't seem to work, don't beat yourself up (as other issues may be at play). The more you stress, the less milk you'll produce. Relax, breathe and continue playing around to find something that works. You got this!

Increase your vitamin intake.

Your body will do what it needs to produce milk and it will pull the necessary nutrients it needs as well. Even if your body is depleted, it will go into fat storage mode to be able to produce the milk baby needs. It can also be extremely hard to ensure your body is receiving all of the nutrients it needs via your diet — especially with sleep deprivation and minimal down time for yourself. Taking iron supplements, increasing your calcium and magnesium intake, or adding fenugreek to your diet may also aid in increasing milk supply. The goal is to replenish your body constantly, to ensure the output isn't depleting your own nutrition.

Reduce alcohol intake (even though beer increased your supply a few times).

You may have heard the story: a mother's milk was low, she drank one beer and like magic her breasts were filled with milk. The truth is that, drinking a beer can in fact increase your milk supply due to the yeast (Brewer's yeast is extremely helpful in increasing supply). But constantly drinking beer (or any alcohol) will eventually reduce your milk supply. Sometimes a quick hit is all you need, but aim to find longer lasting solutions versus short term fixes.

How to Reduce an Oversupply

There are also circumstances where you may need to decrease your milk supply (i.e. when weaning, struggling with frequently clogged milk ducts or mastitis, excessive leaking, letting down too aggressively causing baby to choke, or dealing with loss). Whatever the reason, finding ways to decrease production can be just as beneficial as knowing how to increase production.

The following are some tips to help **reduce milk production**:

- **The use of sage, peppermint and oregano** have been found to adversely impact milk production.

Adding them to your diet may help to reduce your supply.

- **Placing cabbage leaves on your breast** (similar to when your breasts were engorged), helps to decrease milk production. The use of cold compresses in general will help to decrease production and can help relieve any pain associated with the changes to your breast (they may be tender).

- **Allowing your baby to feed from a bottle during some sessions** will help to decrease milk production. NOTE: If you're skipping or lessening your nursing sessions, remember to drain just enough milk from your breasts to avoid developing clogged ducts. The less you remove, the less your body will begin to make, but you don't want to risk developing mastitis in the process.

- **Finding supplements or teas that focus on reducing milk supply** can be extremely effective as well. Many brands that focus on increasing milk supply also provide products that decrease supply as well.

The good news is that whether you're attempting to increase or decrease your supply, there are many ways in which you can go about it. The most important thing to remember is to avoid stress as much as possible. Having a baby is inherently stressful, but things that are completely out of your control and don't serve you or baby well should be released from your psyche. Your body is focused on producing food for baby. The more your stress, the more you divert energy away from your body's priorities.

With a just a bit of research you'll find plenty of other moms are exactly where you are, or have been where you are in your struggles. Don't give up and just allow your body the time it needs to adjust to the huge changes that have and are occurring. Everything doesn't have to happen right away. Give yourself time and with a little patience, you'll be surprised at what magic your body creates.

Freezing Your Milk

It's a powerful tool to freeze excess milk. By simply placing your milk in (or pumping directly into) freezer bags specialized for breastmilk, dating them and throwing them in the freezer, you'll have an incredible storage of antibodies for baby. For example, if baby (or their siblings) gets sick, squirting breastmilk directly into their nose can become one of your greatest aids in treating stuffy noses, colds, viruses, et cetera. If baby experiences a rash, cradle cap, eczema, et cetera, breastmilk can be used as topical solutions. Cooking with your breastmilk (i.e. adding it to baby's purees) will add extra nutrients to their ever-evolving palate.

Freezing your milk from the beginning (and by finding your own rhythm for pumping and storing) will be a great help on those days when you need to be away from baby. The more you store early, the less stressful it can be when it's time to go back to work, enjoy a date night, or enjoy a full night's rest while your spouse offers the bottle. All in all, it can never cause more harm to save your milk. You may also have the ability to donate some to other mothers who may be in need. If your freezer starts to overflow, simply use some of that milk for your older toddler's meals (great addition to smoothies) to give their body's some extra antibodies. The magical powers of breastmilk are just way too good to waste! With breastmilk able to freeze for upwards of 9 months without losing its potency, baby will be able to enjoy the benefits of your breastmilk long after you have made the transition to wean.

Weaning (grab the cabbage)

As aforementioned, there are many ways to aid in reducing milk production. This is especially important to remember when it's time to **wean** baby (transitioning from breastmilk to other liquids, foods, or supplements). The process of weaning varies for everyone. Some do it early, others do it well into the toddler age. Some experience baby led weaning and others must make the decision before their baby is palpably ready. Whatever the case and for whatever reason, when the time is right, you must follow your heart.

Weaning can be an emotional rollercoaster, as you're officially ending one of the most sacred moments of motherhood. It can also be a monumental occasion to celebrate, as you and baby are officially starting a new phase in your relationship. It can be emotional, exciting, sad, great, painful, pain free, a big deal or not. However, it makes you feel is equally as powerful as anyone else's experience. Aside from the special bond you and baby developed, your hormones are drastically changing as your body prepares to stop production altogether. The manner by which you wean can also impact your body's reaction to it (stopping abruptly versus gradually weaning nets a different process). Regardless of the manner by which you wean, below are a few helpful tips to aid in your transition:

Don't concern your process with others.

Deciding to wean is just as personal as deciding to breastfeed in the first place. At the end of the day, the decision is yours because it's your body. You and baby's journey is unique and cannot be compared to anyone else's. One friend may have breastfed for three months while another for 22 months. Regardless, what is right for your journey is personal. People may share their opinions with the best of intentions. Try not to get wrapped up in the opinions or judgments of others. Own your decision and honor yourself for however amount of time you decide to nurse. It's all incredible! Remember that.

Mind your hormonal shifts.

Your body has been operating in a special manner in order to produce milk for baby. Your estrogen has been low, prolactin has been high and your calcium levels have continuously been dropping. Once you stop nursing, your body has to regulate itself. When you wean, the drop in prolactin and oxytocin may make you feel more emotional than you have recently been. That is perfectly normal. If you're sad or depressed, be sure to share your feelings with others. You're not alone and you shouldn't wallow in your emotions. This moment will pass and you'll find happiness in the start of your new journey with baby.

But you must give yourself some time. Some moms start to feel normal again in a couple of weeks, for others it may take months. Just take it day by day. Soon enough, you'll start to remember what it was like to feel like yourself again.

It can be painful (don't get engorged).

It's important to take into account that it will take some time for your breasts to stop producing the milk all together (weeks or months). During this process, it's imperative not to let your breasts become engorged — as you don't want to experience clogged ducts or mastitis. Gradually weaning may be the most preferred method, but for those who must stop abruptly, you can still gradually allow your milk production to halt. Rather than avoiding expressing milk altogether, you may need to express just enough to provide relief, but not too much to encourage more production. Over time, your body will get the memo and you'll get to a point where you no longer have to express anything. Allow your body the time it needs to normalize itself. Remember to add cabbage to your breasts often, use ice packs when necessary and take pain relievers if the pain is unbearable or the tenderness makes it hard to get through the day.

It can also feel like pregnancy (tired, nauseas, dizzy).

One of the least talked about topics regarding weaning is the sickness that may come with it. While some moms may have an easy transition, there are others (like myself) who experience sickness — similar to being pregnant. There are times when weaning may cause bouts of nausea, dizziness, extreme fatigue, irritability and bloating. There are also those who experience a dip in their appetite as their metabolism slows down. If you're someone who experiences this, just know that it too is normal. Soon enough this phase will pass — and within the next couple of weeks you'll feel normal again (respectively). Avoid going too long without eating; incorporate crackers to your diet to help with the nausea; and sleeping if and when you can may help to mitigate the exhaustion (sounds like pregnancy right?). All in all, very soon, you'll have your full body back (in whatever capacity this means for you).

You will have new breasts.

Your breasts have probably been full and voluptuous during this journey. Now that you're weaning, it's likely that they will be smaller — and possibly smaller than before your breastfeeding journey. The good news is that, however your breasts return to form, they did exactly what they were created to do! You brought life into this world and sustained that life with the absolute greatest start you could give. You were the life source of your baby for however amount of time and if your breasts are a little different in shape afterwards, you deserve them! They are exactly what they need to be. And in time, they will take life again. Allow yourself time to heal and recover. Honor your body and your process.

You may actually gain weight (and quickly).

Unbeknownst to many, post weaning, your body is likely to still operate in the same manner it did while breastfeeding — i.e. you may still have the same hunger cues. While nursing, your body burned off approximately 500 more calories than normal. And with the need to produce milk, your metabolism increased as well as your appetite (probably needing a snack before or after each feeding). Though it may seem like a subtle shift in nature, the moment you decide to wean, your eating routine can become gravely evident. When I weaned my son, he was 11 months old and I was 7 months pregnant. Not only was I thoroughly exhausted from a rough pregnancy and nursing simultaneously, but the flavor of my milk changed as my colostrum began to come in. My son no longer liked the taste; thus, weaning was quick (a one day process) and I felt free the moment I stopped. Three months later I was back to breastfeeding. I decided to wean my daughter around 14 months, as I was finally ready.

At that point, I had been nursing for approximately 2.5 years straight — so when I stopped, I was eating as if I were still nursing and burning off those extra 500 calories. Unfortunately, my metabolism slowed way down and I gained 10 pounds in two weeks. I went from feeling great (having worked off most of my baby weight), to a week later, not being able to fit my jeans! With a quick online search, I learned of the norms of weight gain post weaning. My hormones were all over the place, my appetite was changing, my metabolism was basically at a standstill and my body needed time to adjust. It took approximately three months to finally feel like myself again (and for my milk production to fully end).

In hindsight, nursing my babies was completely worth how hard the weaning process was — even though I was miserable during those three months. So, while you may often hear about the perks of dropping those last 10 pounds after weaning or the immediate surge of energy you'll have, remember your regulating hormones and treat yourself accordingly (with patience and compassion). At the end of the day, you'll still look and truly be one fabulous mom.

You will have renewed energy and freedom.

In time, you'll soon have more energy, more calcium going back to your bones and increased freedoms you haven't had in a while! You can drink alcohol or use your herbs again (if you stopped during breastfeeding), you can wear what you want (no more nursing friendly V-necks for a while), and you can be away from baby for longer periods of time! Congratulate yourself, as this is a turning point for you.

It may be hard and emotional at first, but it will absolutely be okay. Whether it was an easy process or lengthy and tiresome, all that matters is that you did it. Everything is a season and once you overcome weaning, there will be another obstacle waiting for you to tackle. You were never going to nurse forever, so celebrate and treat yourself for this milestone you have achieved! You're in a new season and you should be proud.

You did it!!

chapter 12

You Are Not Alone

N o single experience into or throughout motherhood is exactly like another; yet, there are often overflows of commonalties that allow us to find the inspiration, encouragement and hope we need to push through. With this in mind, the upcoming chapters were designed to help with just that — offer information in a way by which you can choose what works best for you and your nuanced journey (entrenched with the constant reminder that you're not alone). You'll learn information you can then put into practice anyway you see fit. If there is something that piques your interest, I implore you to dive further into it. Once you start your researching process, chances are you'll realize just how much more there is to learn.

Talking with other moms can become a saving grace. At times, the simple fact of knowing that someone else is or has experienced your particular hurdle can help mitigate the pain of those hard days (and we all have them). Learning tips and tricks from others can help broaden your thinking on how to efficiently and effectively tackle problems. It's imperative not to judge yourself or others. At the end of the day, we are all just figuring this parenting thing out as we go.

As you heal during your 4th trimester, you must remember that everything is a season. Every baby is different—so don't worry if one thing worked for your first baby but not your second or third. Comparing children can and usually ends up being a recipe for disaster. Monitoring your desires, expectations and milestone mapping will be a great help in finding and maintaining patience. Your baby will feel that sense of love and support, rather than the pressure to be someone they aren't or haven't reached yet. Keep in mind that you and your spouse/partner come first. Above all, you must cherish your relationship and refuse to let that magnetic love go to wayside. That love for each other is essential to your sanity and helps to hold on to the piece of you that should always remain.

It's also imperative to trust your **mommy gut** — your special intuitive power that is instinctual and most times inexplicable. We all have it. During your postpartum recovery, listen to your body and pay attention to your emotions. Recognize all of the thoughts that don't serve you and find ways to let them go. Remember your own brilliance and don't shy away from it. You must fall in love with your mind, your body, your spouse/partner and the journey you have embarked on with your baby. Just having that as a goal, without worrying too much on how to achieve it, can make all the difference in reshaping and revitalizing your habitual thinking. For what we think is a direct reflection of who we are. And who we are will absolutely make shape by the manner in which we parent. It's my hope that the following chapters provide some insight on what you can expect during this 4th trimester and encourage you to fall in love with your newly evolved and empowered self.

nothing is more real than a thought

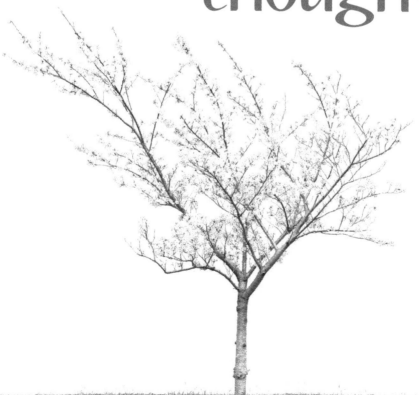

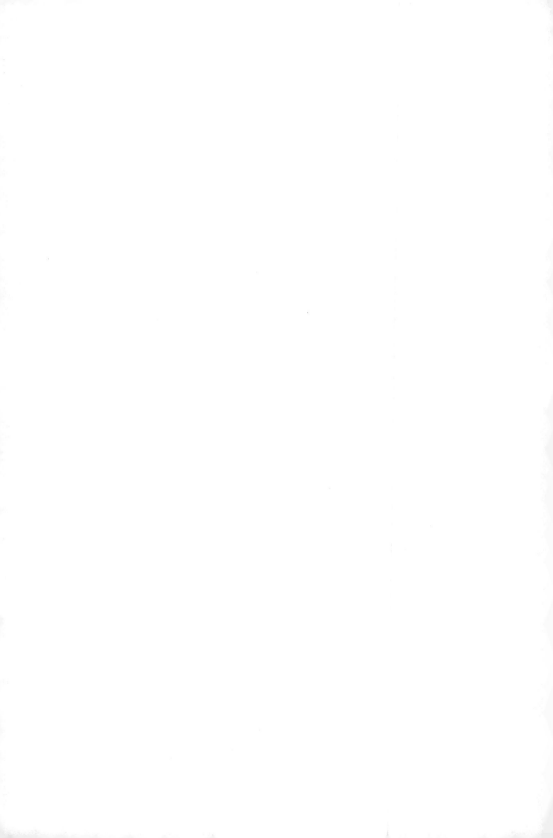

chapter 13

Sleep Deprivation

I t may feel like a tired joke; the one where all parents warn you to get as much asleep as you can before having your baby (in a playful but kind of serious tone). The truth of the matter is this: there is no sleep deprivation like that of having babies. Period. The level of exhaustion at times truly feels unbearable. Some moms may find that having help around the house for a while allows them to sneak in a few naps. But regardless of the circumstances and even with help, it's almost certain that you'll experience some form of sleep deprivation. If not, then keep up whatever you're doing! For the rest of us, there is still hope.

The harsh reality to accept is that, there are hardly any quiet moments of stillness to merely catch up on sleep. Typically, when we finally get our baby down for a nap or bed, it's the first time of the day where we can catch up on life; hence, the importance of finding a schedule and tactics that work for your family. The more sleep you can get as a parent, the better off you'll be (and happier you'll find yourself).

Sleep deprivation effects all parties involved — not just mom. So it's important to remember that everyone is tired (especially in those moments where you want to curse everybody out in the entire house — it happens). There are many reasons why sleep escapes us as new moms. A few include (but definitely aren't limited to):

- excitement of finally holding our baby

- nerves and adrenaline (whether from your birthing experience or simply holding baby in your arms)

- constantly checking on baby (whereas some moms can sleep while their baby is sleeping, there are others who can't get past the nerves and monitor their baby)

- feeding throughout the night (and day)—always feeding and never resting can cause a gargantuan shift in our sleep cycles, making it harder to fall and stay asleep

- crying (or any sounds for that matter) that our babies make

- simply trying to adjust and figure out life with a new person involved who is completely dependent upon you, making it hard to find a great night's sleep

- trying to have a life outside of merely parenting can make it hard to find sleep too—as you try to find a balance between parenting and still doing things that are fun and make you laugh (babies aside)

- the lack of downtime (parenting is 24/7—no breaks)

- feeling overwhelmed and stressed can painfully affect our inability to sleep (less sleep equals more stress, more stress equals less sleep—a cyclical issue)

- trying to balance work and parenting (especially with a fully dependent newborn and accident-prone toddlers)

- a lack of a support system can make it impossible to find sleep—where there is no help, there is no moment to regroup and rest

As any parent can tell you, the list of reasons why it's almost impossible to come up on great sleep with newborns is endless. Giving encouraging words to other parents with babies and toddlers is a great way to simply connect with other parents struggling with sleep — and offers a brief moment to laugh about how hard parenting is. Talk with other parents. We're all sleepy — trust me.

Trying to cope with sleep deprivation is another full-time job. And it's important to understand how that lack of sleep can impact our bodies and our psyche. Some of these effects include, but are not limited to:

- harboring negative emotions (that could result in hostility and resentment)

- depression (particularly postpartum depression, which is discussed in a later chapter)

- reduces cognitive function (creates problems with memory, problem solving, fast reaction time, et cetera)
- can cause weight gain (slowing down of our metabolism)

The purpose of sharing the impact of sleep deprivation is not to scare you into feeling that the things aforementioned are absolutely going to happen. The goal is to help better prepare you, so when you find yourself feeling intense emotions you cannot explain, you may be able to take a step back and recognize the immense emotional drainage that a lack of sleep causes. This may allow you the ability to recognize when to ask for help in order to regroup and find yourself a much-needed nap. Whatever the case, it's my desire to encourage honesty with yourself and your support system.

There is no single parent who can successfully parent alone. We all have help and we all have moments when we must rely on help to make it through the day. Sleep deprivation is real and the effects so quantifiable that it's imperative to be able to recognize the signs. Fortunately, there are some things you can do to combat these side effects.

Stop beating yourself up.

To be clear, parenting is not always a walk in the park. It can get hard and messy and that is okay. It's imperative that you constantly remind yourself that every baby is different, every experience is different and at the end of the day, we're ALL just figuring this thing out as we go! Stop feeling pressure to always explain or defend yourself to others. You spend enough energy all day and night trying to comfort baby — reserve the rest of that energy for treating and loving on yourself. No single parent has perfected parenting and there is no "one size fits all" handbook.

The more people scrutinize and judge, the more likely they're pushing their insecurities onto you via their ego. Ignore anything that doesn't serve you during this time and don't apologize for doing what you need to do to get sleep (even if that means missing a few events). Friends and family will be fine and tend to understand that you can't be everywhere all the time. The more you let go of unnecessary pressures of perfection, the more you can find peace. When you find peace, your body and mind can relax and you can find sleep (eventually).

Try and sleep whenever you can.

You'll hear it often, but it's true: laundry, dishes and cleaning can wait! In the first months of baby's arrival, the most important thing to do is to find a rhythm that works for the household. In time, as baby starts to adjust to life outside of the womb, you'll be able to find your way into completing all of those chores. Essentially, the immediate goal is to find as much peace, serenity and sleep as humanly possible. If going to bed with a messy kitchen is completely out of the question, then ask for help. Ask for someone to help you with cleaning the kitchen so you can get rest and have your peace of mind. If vacuuming is therapeutic for you (everyone is different), then do what you need to do to help clear your mind.

The more you can find peace internally, the more peace that will permeate into your external. Do what you must, but make sleep a priority — for a clean house, but a sleep deprived parent isn't the win we all need. The stronger you feel, the better you can attack each day. *(Remember, if you start doing chores during every nap, your body will get tired as soon as baby wakes up! It's almost nature's way of punishing us for not taking advantage of the downtime. So relax!)*

Establish a schedule.

It will take some time and patience, but the short-term sacrifice of figuring out a schedule for baby will produce massive long-term gains. Babies / toddlers love predictability—it represents safety and stability. Establishing a routine (whether soft or rigid) can help you plan your days more effectively and can be helpful when trying to plan a day / night away. For example, offering your babysitter a mock schedule of the day will ensure that baby sleeps and eats on time.

Most importantly, the more established your schedule, the more sleep baby will get. Tired babies are often cranky and moody and it makes it extremely hard to learn and focus (just like adults). Sleep deprivation for babies can also have a grave impact on their developmental growth. So, establishing some sort of schedule can pay huge dividends for everyone. Remember that, even a flexible schedule is better than no schedule. Allowing baby to find a routine can help make bedtime much easier and, in the end, can help you get more sleep as well (that's the goal!). More on schedules in the next chapter.

Stop obsessing over parenting "rules".

Parenting books, websites, forums and advice from others can become extremely overwhelming. The more we stress over finding perfection as parents, the less likely we are to allow things to happen organically. The more we decide to abide by very stringent timelines established by some person we will never meet, the harder the overall experience. Sometimes it's best to let our babies decide when they're ready to transition to different things.

Not every baby needs to ditch their pacifier at six months — some babies may not want to start solid foods until 9 months — some babies may not have any interest in potty training until three years old — some babies may be more interested in cognitive development then physical (or vice versa). The point is, the more we stress over perfection based on a subjective and highly imperfect system, the more unnecessary stress we add to our plates. The more stress, the less sleep. The less sleep, the more stress. The less we obsess over things that aren't really problems, the more we can enjoy the beauty of motherhood. The less we force our babies/toddlers to do things because we are socially embarrassed by the opinions of the others, the happier our babies will be and the happier we will be. Breathe. You're doing just fine. And baby loves you for it.

Take a walk and take care of your body.

Sometimes you (and maybe baby) just need a burst of fresh air. Being stuck in the house all the time can drive you crazy. Taking a walk, which can become your form of exercise, can actually help you feel more energized. By moving your body, it may help you sleep better. Going outside, getting fresh air and moving your body, are all things that can help get you relaxed and renewed. Also, adding vitamins such as magnesium to your diet, or adding lavender to your pillow case at night may help to calm you down before bed.

Have someone else hold your baby.

If and when you find yourself completely upset (with baby, or with yourself), you should ask for help. There are times when you rock baby to sleep for two hours, only to have them wake up after 30 minutes. There are times when you've finally got baby down to sleep and some random noise wakes them up, starting your process all over again. <u>There are times, when we must be honest with ourselves and recognize that we are too upset to hold our baby.</u> Our energy directly impacts theirs. The more honest we can be with our vulnerability in this time, the more peace we can find. The more peace we find, the better our ability to find good sleep. Sometimes you'll just need a nap, but sometimes you'll simply need a couple minutes to just breathe and regroup. Don't feel bad about this — ask for your nap, take the time for yourself and try to remember how blessed you are (even when you haven't slept for three weeks straight).

Put your phone down.

Drop the habit of looking at your phone before bed (and so much during the day). Being more present during the day can help you find more efficient ways of parenting and taking care of yourself. Ridding of the phone at night will also help to regulate your melatonin levels. With too much light, our serotonin levels increase and our bodies start to wake up (confusing our internal clocks). When you keep it dark, melatonin is released and you can find it easier to fall asleep.

Find the best way to establish strong sleeping habits (sleep training isn't for everyone).

It's also imperative that we stop driving ourselves crazy over sleep training books, methods, et cetera. Yes, babies need sleep; but not all babies find that sleep using sleep training methods. Around the world, most babies sleep with or in the same room as their parents. The Westernized societal customs of rushing babies into their own rooms, isn't always necessary or beneficial for every family.

Each baby is different and will adjust to sleeping differently. Trying different methods (including varied sleep training styles) is helpful, but becoming stressed when a certain method doesn't work will make the process longer and harder. Babies who sleep with or in the same room as their parents experience unique benefits than those who sleep independently early on:

- They typically aren't sleep deprived (which is helpful for parents trying to get sleep as well).

- Babies don't develop psychological scars or abandonment issues from being left in a foreign space crying for long periods of time (*NOTE: If the cry it out method works for you, then do it! Don't judge your process.*)

- These babies can be nursed or rocked back to sleep and continue sleeping throughout the night

While some babies may relish in the aforementioned benefits, there may be some babies who just enjoy their own space. The point is that all babies are different, and not allowing baby to find their best means of sleeping due to social pressures and judgment will only make it harder for you to find sleep.

Your focus should simply be on finding what gets you the most sleep and to just do it. Do what you need to do. If baby needs a pacifier, then give it to them. (*Note: You've likely never seen a 10-year old with a pacifier, so relax—they won't have it forever, but they may need it for a while.*) If they were sleeping alone in their room and then all of a sudden want to cuddle, then let them. Sometimes babies/toddlers go through phases (either emotional or developmental phases). The easier they sleep, the more sleep you get. If you need the baby in your room, great. If you need the baby out of your room, great. There is no single solution. Stop pressuring yourself due to others opinions. Just do you and find sleep however you can.

chapter 14

Postnatal Insomnia

Postpartum sleep deprivation is real and unlike any other level of exhaustion we've likely to have experienced. Insomnia (the inability to fall asleep even when the opportunity presents itself) is also another real and painful component of motherhood many of us face. It's estimated roughly 60% of women between 32 weeks gestation and 8 weeks postpartum experience postnatal insomnia to some degree.[7]

There are numerous reasons why moms find it hard to sleep. Some include:

- trauma from delivery
- fear/paranoia
- excitement or extreme shock
- staying up all night with baby (negatively impacting the circadian rhythm)

- stress

While you may write off your insomnia, it's possible that you may be experiencing clinical insomnia, which significantly increases your chances of developing postpartum depression. In many cases, the intensity of the shock sent to our bodies post-delivery creates the perfect storm for postnatal insomnia. Some triggers may include:

- the major drop in your hormones (more on this in the *Hormones* chapter)

- quantifiable changes in the brain (i.e. your brain rewiring itself to be more alert and sensitive to the sounds of baby)

- intense hot flashes and night sweats (making it impossible to sleep)

- the quick shift in your body clock

- the inability to fall asleep after baby (especially after night wakings/feedings)

- having too much light at night (confusing your internal clock)

One of the most important things to remember when suffering from insomnia, is to try and relax the mind. Instead of attempting to "force" yourself to sleep — which is extremely hard and most times ineffective — start with a change in environment. Now is the time to try switching things up, to make it more conducive to relaxing your spirit. Some examples include playing soft music, using a chargeable candle to change the diaper in the middle of the night versus the huge bright light, reading a book, meditating by closing your eyes during nursing versus staring at your phone, et cetera. By changing your habits, you are allowing yourself the ability to simply get sleepy. The key: you must ask for help when you finally get sleepy (which you will). You must try, if possible, to take advantage of your tiredness. Take the time to sleep (or nap), or even just lay in the bed. Eventually, your body will accept how exhausted you are and give in.

Anxiety is one of the greatest factors that contributes to postnatal insomnia. An article from a great site called Mom Junction offers wonderful tips on how to best combat your insomnia.8 With each tip they've offered, I've added some words of encouragement to help you through:

Sleep when the baby sleeps. This may be hard but try anyways. This will be helpful until your body adjusts to you sleeping less (eventually you'll find a routine and six hours of sleep will actually feel good). Just hang in there and try to relax as much as possible when they sleep — even if that means simply laying down and kicking your feet up.

Go to bed early. Even if you can't go to sleep early every night, allow yourself time for your body to recoup. Enjoy nights of doing nothing. You'll appreciate it and your mind and body (and sleep) will too.

Share the workload. You don't have to do everything. When you want or need help, ask for it.

Try to understand baby's sleep patterns. The more predictable baby's routine, the more predictable the time frames whereby you can rest. Babies/toddlers thrive on consistency. It represents safety and security. It's also calming for them. The calmer they are, the calmer you are — the more sleep you can get.

Create your stress-free zone. Create your space. It's as vital as any other component of motherhood. Without your sanity, nothing else will work. Without sleep, you'll never find your sanity.

Reduce your caffeine intake. As much as you can.

Turn off electric devices before bed. Too much light at night reduces your melatonin (the hormone that makes you sleepy) and increases serotonin (the hormone that wakes you up in the mornings). The more light you have at night, the less your body is able to get sleepy and ready for bed. Relax your mind and your eyes. Put down the phone and allow yourself to get sleepy and actually fall sleep.

Find meditation techniques that work for you. This could include a yoga class, a walk outside, or laying on the couch with relaxing music. Your options are vast and you may need to try different techniques to find the one that works best for you.

Enjoy relaxing teas. (ie: lavender, chamomile, sleepy time teas, etc)

Invest in a massage, chiropractic work, or acupuncture. You may be struggling to sleep due to pain or simply your body being out of whack (don't take for granted how hard it's on your body to look down all day long to nurse, change diapers, talk to baby, et cetera). Sometimes a simple adjustment or massage can go a long way. Our bodies are impacted by the manner in which our spine is in alignment. The stronger our bodies, the better it will respond to the things we need it to do (i.e. sleep).

Communicating your struggles with sleep is essential to not losing your mind. Don't give up on yourself and know that you're not alone. Most mothers experience this at some point during their journey—so your feelings of isolation or as though you aren't normal can be combated in knowing that you aren't now nor will you be alone in this struggle. Having insomnia does not mean you're a bad mom, or inadequate in your journey into motherhood—in fact the opposite is true. Your desire to be your best is nothing to be ashamed of. But if your search for perfection in motherhood negatively impacts your ability to sleep, you must be honest with yourself and adjust accordingly. And never be ashamed to speak up about your struggles. It's imperative and could be your life saver.

Understanding what's really happening to our bodies when we respond to normal situations adversely (i.e. crying hysterically because you can't find the match to a sock), can be a tremendous aid in instilling a greater sense of control and normalcy. Remember the season, try to relax and work on trying new things to create new outcomes that you desire.

chapter 15

Schedules

We may be able to intellectualize the benefits of establishing a schedule, but creating one and sticking to it is a completely different story. Creating a schedule requires a lot of sacrifice (and a lot of missed events). It's inevitable. Fortunately, the long-term benefits gravely outweigh the sacrifices in the short term. It's important to keep in mind that when you develop your schedule you must stick with it. Deviation from the schedule just makes it harder on baby; thus, making it harder on you. As they get older, more flexibility will arise — but setting a strong foundation with established schedules (flexible or fixed) will be your saving grace.

First and foremost, when you develop your schedule never apologize for it. The early months with baby is not the time to please people. It's purely about survival! If you have found baby's schedule and it works for you and your family, nothing is more important. If a friend or family member has an event, but it conflicts with baby's nap or bedtime schedule, skip it (unless you find a baby sitter — in that case, a night out can do you good!). Keep in mind, if a super flexible, noncommittal schedule works for you and your family, then by all means, please ignore this section. It's simply a means to help make life easier. If it doesn't, then skip it.

Only apply what works for you and your family. Remember that your newly established schedule is just for a season. You won't be missing events forever. The truth is that the sacrifices you make now to stay inside and ensure that baby is getting the proper rest they need, will eventually lead to you getting more sleep! Don't let anyone make you feel bad for working your schedule. Your schedule is your helpmate. Soon enough, baby will be sleeping, schedules will be second nature and something else will come up! It's a never-ending cycle, but seasons do end before another starts. Find gratefulness in this time. The less time you have to be out at the events, the more time you get to spend on empowering your dreams, goals and newly evolved self.

chapter 16

How Not to Lose Yourself in Motherhood

One area of motherhood I've found to be the most empowering (and subconscious) is the impact it has on identity. While some moms organically find a perfect harmony between motherhood and their dreams, for the majority, it becomes easy to get completely lost in the world of our babies. Our intrinsic nature to become all consumed with our babies is one of our greatest assets; but also one of the most impacting components that often leads to a complete loss of identity (cue postpartum depression).

The tricky part is discovering how to accept and embrace this new way of life rather than fighting to hold on to the past. The truth is that your priorities will change. Your level of freedom and independence will have to adjust accordingly. Your emotional stability will alter. The feeling of inclusion is often tossed by the wayside. Though bringing forth life is an honor, we would do ourselves a disservice to act as if it doesn't come with an extremely hard wall of adversity to overcome (most of which is contingent upon the power of our thoughts).

For starters, it's imperative we rewire our perspective on the new life we have been thrust into. It can be extremely ease to lose sight of your dreams, fun hobbies, feeling sexy, included, important, loved — falling into a trap of feeling isolated and lonely. The change of going from childless to motherhood is more drastic than words can describe. It rocks your world to the core. Yet, the more you can hold on to things that make you feel like your best self, without finding yourself stuck in a desire for reliving the past, the stronger you can be in your quest to be whole — without losing your identity.

The more empowered your thoughts prior to motherhood, the stronger your propensity to learn and develop even stronger thoughts to combat the negative ones. Holding on to things that make you feel normal is imperative — but they must be in the realm of realistic expectations. For example, you should not expect to make all of the dinner parties like you did in the past. You should not expect to be able to just get up and go somewhere when you feel like it. (*NOTE: Simply trying to walk out of the door will always be an adventure from here on out*). But there are activities you can embrace which may seem small at first, yet with motherhood, can make all the difference between losing your mind and embracing your newly evolved self. Some include but are not limited to:

Date Night

Date night is especially important **within the first month postpartum** if you are physically capable. When baby arrives, it almost feels like time has stopped. That time warp is beautiful bliss, until real life starts to hit. Within the first four weeks post-delivery, you must remind yourself that you're still a whole human being—and that motherhood is an added bonus to who you already were. You cannot forego the things that made you smile in the first place. Don't underestimate the power of a date with your spouse or significant other. You must be careful not to turn a blind eye on each other, which is a subtle yet monumental stance to take. Dates are necessary and the positive magnitude it has in regaining the spark you both had before the baby arrived will set a strong foundation moving forward.

Be Pampered

Whether you're someone who loves getting pampered or not, the feeling of simply having someone take care of you (even if just for a little while) can make all the difference to your sanity. Finding time to just be alone has gargantuan effects on the psyche. Getting your hair done, nails done, a massage, et cetera. is imperative to refocusing and re-energizing your spirit. No matter how silly it may seem, treat yourself. You need it, you deserve it and you'll be so happy you did.

Napping

Sometimes we lose ourselves in the sleep deprivation. Not getting sleep, unable to focus and feeling lost can have a significant impact on our feelings towards ourselves. The less control we feel like we have, the more frazzled and stressed we become. The more we can purposely allow time to take its course, provide ourselves time to physically heal, focus on mentally and emotionally adjusting to our new lifestyles and choosing to be patient with ourselves, the more in control of our thoughts we will be. Something as simple as laying in bed and taking a nap can truly help to rejuvenate your mind, body and spirit. Don't underestimate the resilience it takes to constantly be on the go (especially with your personal needs in last place). It's okay to put yourself first. In fact, the more you take care of yourself, the better equipped you'll be to take care of everyone else.

Exercise

Time away from the baby to get your body moving is one of the greatest ways in which you can start to fall in love with yourself again. Releasing some tension, letting go of old energy, refreshing your body with new oxygen and having some time to sweat is incredible in your search to loving your new place in life. Now that your priority is always on baby, it can be hard to find the energy to do anything for yourself that is worthwhile. The truth is, the more you can find time to work out, the more energy you'll have — and energy is the one thing we all need more of during this time.

Girls Day / Girls Night

Becoming a mom doesn't mean you're no longer allowed to have fun. There may be limitations on how many events you can attend, but it doesn't take away from how fly, fresh, fun and funky you were before motherhood. It's not a rule that once you have kids you must become dull and inactive. You must have fun in ways you did before. You must hold somethings dear to you that you did prior to motherhood in a means of not losing yourself completely. You're not the same, but doing things that are fun (just for you) is essential to your well-being. You're allowed to have fun, so go do it! Even if you know you have to rush home before the little one is up for a night time feed, sometimes it's worth being extremely tired the next day. It's not every day, so enjoy yourself and laugh!

Recreate Your Vision Board

The most important component to not losing yourself completely in motherhood is never letting go of your ability to dream. Your dreams may change, but you must always have a dream. You must have something (aside from your children) that gets you up and out of bed in the morning. You must have something that gives you butterflies. You must have something that your mind drifts to in those late nights when you're rocking a crying baby alone in a dark room. You must have thoughts that get you excited. You must continue or start dreaming. And it must be big dreams.

Every day of motherhood presents a new hurdle to overcome — and so many moms find nuanced and unique ways to do that. If your passion is to help other moms, then do it! If you now have a dream to create children's books, then do it! If you have a dream that has absolutely nothing to do with mothers or children, then do it! You must have a dream, because it's the one thing that will keep you going when all else feels out of whack. Parenting comes with a ton of ups and downs. One day baby is sleeping for 10 hours straight and the next, they're up five times a night. It happens. Life happens. And when it does, something must organically and intensely put you back on track.

Something must get your feet going, so you can be excited about just being you. And the magnitude of your motivation cannot be contingent upon your environment. You must find a dream, a powerful thought, that is more magnanimous than your circumstances. Something that you can revert to when baby is crying, nipples are sore, body is fatigued, and your sense of self is dwindling. Find that source that brings you back to you. And that source starts with a thought. Remember, there is nothing more real in life than a thought. Ignite your perspective, and keep dreaming. And most importantly, believe without a shadow of a doubt that you can achieve every goal you set. If you recreate your vision board and don't believe wholeheartedly that those dreams will manifest, then you've simply made a poster. And you my dear are much more capable and closer to your dreams than you know.

You'll always be a mom, so it's okay (and necessary) to do things that simply make you happy. You need this. And the example you will set, and the foundation by which you raise your children, will manifest in the lives you change. You got this!

Tell Yourself How Incredible You Are

Now that you're a mom, you have more to fight for. When we lose our identity, we lose the thing that we we're fighting for. When we fall into a monotonous routine and never allow ourselves nuanced experiences, we become the opposite of what we were designed to do: which is to create. We are creative beings by nature and we were created to constantly evolve. Thus, when this massive change impacts our lives, we must allow our dreams and goals to evolve as well.

You must do whatever makes you feel like yourself, in the realm of responsibility for your baby. It takes work and is a huge learning curve; but overtime (with persistence and patience), you'll find the right balance. Wrapped in the spit up clothes, sweats, messy hair and sloppy days, is still the vibrant, sexy, fun and fearless YOU. If dressing up every now and again makes you feel normal, do it! Do what speaks to your heart and don't judge it. Being "selfish" isn't inherently a bad thing, especially when rooted in honest self love. Selfishness only becomes a deterrent when ego gets involved — because ego is simply an overcompensation of our insecurities. The more we hold on to what we love about ourselves, the less insecurities we harbor and the more our "selfishness" becomes rooted in simple sanity and peace of mind (versus abandoning our responsibilities as parents). Taking care of ourselves does not equate to flopping on the job. The opposite is true. The better you feel, the stronger you can be for your children and your family. Never, ever, ever, neglect yourself.

A few other reasons why we may start to lose our sense of identity within motherhood include:

- solely focusing on our babies

- forgetting to care about our appearance

- never having a second of stillness — always on the move, but never doing anything for ourselves

- priorities have completed shifted (i.e. kids over career)

- we have lost our freedoms

As we know, the stronger our thoughts, the more empowered our perspective and the better our outcomes will be (especially in establishing the foundation of parenting). With time, you'll be able to recognize the things you need to incorporate into your new schedule in order to feel whole and human. A few important reminders as you embark on this journey of self-love, awareness and care:

Stop Comparing Yourself and Your Baby

The more time spent looking at others and comparing yourself and your situation (whether consciously or subconsciously), the less likely it is you'll ever find the peace of mind you so desperately need. Your motherhood journey will be unlike anyone else's because your baby is unlike anyone else's. Though our experiences may have parallel paths (and there are struggles we need to talk with other moms about), there are some things that don't require you to observe others. The more you spend time looking at other moms either in public or online, the less energy you can exert into uplifting yourself and your children. Regardless of what you see, everyone is going through something. Don't wish to have anyone else's situation. You're exactly where you're supposed to be and your baby chose you for a reason. Honor that.

Stop Judging Yourself

Stop being so hard on yourself. Just do your best. That's all any parent has ever done in the history of parenting. That's all we can do. No single person has perfected parenting because no single approach works for everyone. Each person we raise in this world will create their own reality based on the thoughts in their own minds. The more we set out to simply offer the greatest start for our babies and stop striving for perfection (which doesn't exist by the way), the more free we can feel. We must help them seek purpose over perfection, and we must allow ourselves room to make mistakes and learn in order to do that. The more we can smile and be grateful for what we do have, rather than focusing on all the things we wished we had, the less we will judge ourselves. For it's important to remember that there are so many women who would do anything to be in our very position. We must not squander it by being ungrateful and beating ourselves up. Our faith and our gratefulness shows in our self-love. So, love on yourself hard and apply your faith.

Find What Makes You Feel Beautiful

Play around until you find things that make you happy, feel beautiful and bring fun into your life. Our babies are all of those things, but you're still your own light being that has needs specially tailored towards you. Take time and make time to discover what makes you fall in love with yourself again. The more you can love yourself, the more you can love the greatest extension of yourself.

Laugh

One of the coolest things about the power of the mind is that we can convince ourselves of any reality we choose. Our brain doesn't distinguish the difference between a fake laugh or a real one. Once you laugh, oxytocin is released through your body. Which means, even the start of a fake laugh can make you feel better. Even if you feel like there is nothing to laugh about, just laugh. It will make you feel better and give your spirit a moment of pause and release — helping put things into perspective and remind you of just how blessed you are. Laughing helps us to remember this moment is just a season and it will be gone soon enough. Rather than wishing we could go back in time, our goal should be to appreciate each stage of motherhood more profoundly. Laughter can be a way to bring you back to your happy place and into a more empowered space.

Drop the Guilt

This is so important, there is an entire chapter dedicated to it! Next up...

chapter 17

Drop the Guilt

T his is a line I've heard my own mom inspire so many other moms with. An avid mentor to all she comes in contact with, I can honestly say I've truly learned how to be my greatest self as a light being, woman, wife and mother by simply watching her in action. One of her greatest character strengths is her ability to drop the guilt. She had me at a very young age, never breast-fed once, worked up until she gave birth via emergency cesarean section and was back at work a few weeks later because she had to be.

Both she and my dad worked full time jobs and it was the only reality I knew. My mom travelled a lot with work; thus, she couldn't make every basketball game or school performance and even missed a few birthdays. Essentially, the very things most of us choose to beat ourselves up about, were the same things she chose to cut herself slack on. The moment she dropped the guilt of not being able to be everywhere and do everything, she was free. The moment she became free, so did I. The funniest part is, she was so free from guilt, that I don't ever remember her not being there. Even if she wasn't, I don't have a single memory of feeling abandoned or unloved.

The truth is we cannot be everywhere at all times, or everything for everybody. It's not only impossible, but it's ineffective. The more we stretch ourselves thin, the less of an impact we can make. No matter your journey, whether you're a mom who stays at home with your babies, or works away from home, to some degree we all find ways to feel inadequate in our role as moms. No matter how much we invest into our babies, there is always room to do more — and we never feel like we've done enough to fill that void. The honesty we must implore upon ourselves is that, we are enough and we are doing enough. Our babies will be just fine!

With all of the love and attention we place on our babies, sometimes it's easy to miss out on just how resilient they are. Our job as parents is not to be perfect versions of some fantasy we have crafted in our heads. Our jobs are simply to lay the strongest foundation for our children to thrive and make an impact on this world. Our children will not hate us for following our dreams, even if it means not being there for every single milestone or event. If we love them unconditionally and are there for them, that is all they will hold in their own hearts. But if we have animosity, anger, or regret in our hearts from having children and throwing away our dreams, it will show and they will feel it.

No amount of money can replace time spent with our babies — but no amount of regret is worth giving up on your dreams in pursuit of a false reality of parenthood. No parent can be present for every single thing for every single child — and if so, something has been sacrificed (and that usually expresses itself in some form of placing themselves on the back-burner). Sacrifice in the short term is beneficial for long term gain. But giving up altogether for the sake of never missing anything is too heavy of a weight to carry. You must do things that fulfill your spirit and you must not feel guilty about it!

If you aren't fully committed to your personal hopes and dreams, you're not doing what you were designed to do. If you're unhappy, you can't parent the way you truly want to. The more moms you talk to, the more likely you'll find that you're not alone in your quest for harmony. People without children may be able to intellectualize what you're going through, but it's through experiential knowledge and wisdom from those who have gone through or are going through it, that can help bring you the encouragement and insight your heart needs. Something very important to remember if you start to feel guilty about doing something for yourself, that may cost you a missed moment: **proximity isn't effective if you are emotionally withdrawn, psychologically vacant, or spiritually depleted.** The more well-rounded you are, the better you can parent. Effective parenting is only plausible with self-love and self-care. And each mom has different needs to fulfill that necessity. Whatever that is for you, don't judge it. Embrace it and drop the guilt!

Don't judge your situation, your choices, your needs, or your dreams. You must appreciate your uniqueness and solely focus on ways to harmonize the best parts of yourself, your dreams and your family. You have what you need for baby— that's why they chose you. If baby feels loved, whether you work, stay home, or work from home, they will thrive. Your baby will remember how you made them feel and that will set the foundation for their outlook on life (which will create their reality). They won't remember if you missed the first time they tried avocado because you had to work. But they will remember just how exciting it is to be in mommy's arms and that's what matters. They won't remember every time you weren't there, but they will always remember that you were. They will know they're loved, because you're fully capable of loving them—and that's only when you truly love yourself.

Remember, at the end of the day, you are adequate. No single person has it all figured out. Drop the guilt because it doesn't serve anyone. Feeling guilty about missing something doesn't magically make the time go backwards and allow you to be there. There are going to be so many milestones and moments that you have witnessed and that you will in the future. Don't beat yourself up. Remember what you're working towards and remember your greatest inspirations. Your baby will be the ultimate motivator—and no single person can stop you from achieving your dreams with that amount of resiliency. For baby's sake, your dreams will get done. And they will love you for being their greatest example of going after your heart's desires. As my mom always tells me: **you were created for this moment and you are MORE than enough**.

chapter 18

Overcoming Fear

Becoming a parent is scary. It's scary to have to be responsible for another human being, when it's hard enough taking care of ourselves. The great news is that, as our ancestors before us, we always figure out a way to evolve and embrace our ability to raise up the next generation. Even with nerves or anxieties about parenting, we must not ever allow ourselves to become paralyzed by fear. You'll do great and so will baby. Just do your absolute best—that's all that is required (everything incredible with motherhood falls in line with this premise). Your best self in parenting is not the convenient version of your best, but actively seeking to become the best fulfillment of who you were created to be — no matter what.

As a divine creation, you're able to plant anything you want in your mind. And whatever you plant, you undoubtedly produce. Period. There is no deviation from this law. Are you planting fruit or poison? The manifestation of your life and how you feel are your greatest indicators of this. You cannot produce both: only fruit or only poison (poisonous fruit is still poison). However you mentally embrace your journey into and throughout motherhood journey will be your outcome. You create your own reality simply by the thoughts you allow to consume your mind. Your baby is coming into your world — you set the tone, you lay the foundation and you have the final say in what that will be. The great news is that, no matter where you currently are, you're fully capable of evolving your mind and elevating how you see yourself.

One of the greatest ways in which you can retrain poisonous thoughts is by solely focusing on what you want (refusing to exert any effort in rehashing all of the things you fear or don't have). Focusing on fear will cause that to permeate your reality. You must exert energy solely into your hopes, dreams and exciting moments you'll have during this journey. Envision the best case scenario and work towards that. If you dull down your "best case scenario" (i.e. your dreams) to something that feels more feasible and within your reach, it can indicate a lack of faith. Your dreams are a direct reflection of how strong your faith is. And fear (lack of faith) is the only thing that can stop your dreams from becoming your reality.

Remember that fear itself is not a real, tangible thing. The feelings produced are a result of those thoughts, but they are essentially self-created thoughts we have allowed to become habitual — thus, establishing our belief system. Internal peace does not require any changes to our external situations. Positivity requires an external shift to create internal happiness — but **powerful thoughts** are what create the peace within that will shift your life in ways you never imagined. And this can happen with your baby here! Your dream is not taken off the table because you're a parent. Your baby is not a deterrent, but rather your greatest reason why. Don't be fearful. Have faith and create the life you want—for your sake and for theirs.

it's all good

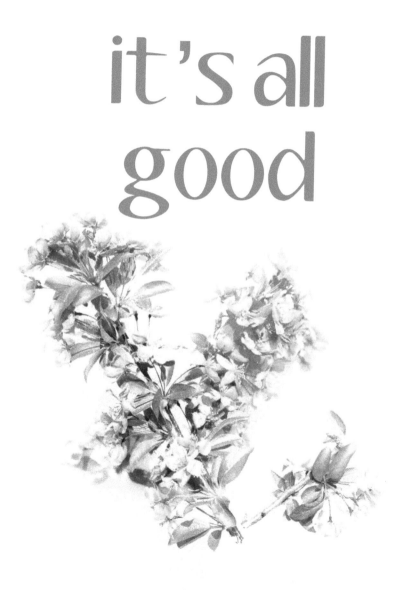

chapter 19

Finding Yourself Again (Self Love + Confidence)

L ife happens. Even with all of the knowledge at your fingertips and an acute awareness for your mental and emotional well-being, you may look up one day to find that you have in fact lost yourself. And that's okay. You aren't the first and surely won't be the last. Take a deep breath and regroup. Revisit the information you already know and be honest with yourself on where you are in comparison to where you want to be.

Reimagining the vision board will always be a great tool in your arsenal — regardless of when you do it or how many times it changes. But the most important component to remember is that, your vision board is only helpful if you actually believe the things on your vision board will happen. If you have doubt, it's simply an arts and craft project. We must get out of our own way and fall into an empowered place. Before we can dream anything, we must find ourselves worthy of attaining it. If we have any doubt, that energy is permeated into the universe and you'll continue down the same path you're currently on. I'll tell you like my husband tells me: **you must do what you've never done in order to get what you've never had.** If your thoughts are the same, nothing new will emerge. If your doubt is still there, your dreams will not materialize. If you've never had what you truly wanted, it's time to try something new. So, before you create your new vision board, you must get your mind right. One way that may help…

Hello, Hello 30 Day Challenge to Loving Yourself

Get yourself a brand new journal or notebook (size doesn't matter). For 30 consecutive days, write one full page of everything you love about yourself. What you write down doesn't matter, so don't judge anything as irrelevant. For example, *"I love my legs"* is just as important as writing *"I love my compassion"*. Every single thing you love about yourself is important for this test. In the beginning it may seem silly, or hard to find a page full of things that you love. But do it anyway. Don't repeat anything on the same page. And you cannot skip a day. If you do, start over.

In an age where rehashing our past and psychoanalyzing why we feel the way we do about every single thing is the norm, it has become common place to remain fixated with the past.

Understanding why we view the world one way is important when trying to evolve, but reliving and reevaluating those reasons over and over does not add anything powerful to your life. The more we consciously choose to focus on who we want to be, where we want to go and what we want to do, the more those dreams will become reality. There is no other option. Wherever we place our thoughts will manifest in our lives.

The goal is to rewire your brain. By retraining your thoughts, you'll become more conscious of how many negative thoughts you have about yourself on a daily basis. The more we tell ourselves how much we love ourselves, the more we will believe it. And this new habit of thinking will develop into a full-blown belief system — and our beliefs dictate our reality. We see whatever we believe. The more we tell ourselves that we love ourselves, the better we will feel. The better we feel, the more we will love ourselves. The more we can do both, the more abundant and incredible our motherhood journey will be as well. Our brains don't know the difference between real life and a dream. Whatever it harbors, is real. This test is the start to empowering your thoughts and rewiring your brain.

During these 30 days, you will also embark on a 30 day social media detox. The goal here is to encourage complete focus on yourself and everything you're grateful for. A few things will happen:

You will have a lot more time in your day.

The moment you get off of social media, you'll realize just how much time you spend and lose by scrolling and focusing on other people's lives. Whatever your reason for using it, the detox will net you more time. You'll find creative ways to fill your time. And when you have any moments of silence and stillness, you can appreciate them and use them for yourself. Instead of logging online first thing in the morning or last thing before bed, meditate, read a book, write, or study a topic you don't know much about. Learn about the power of your mind. Once you read one article, I promise you won't stop. Whatever you do, don't spend any time on social media. Use all of your time to empower your thoughts. Write in your journal for your 30-day challenge and take back the lost time in your life.

You'll immediately eradicate comparisons.

It's simple: the less you look at others, the less you'll compare yourself to others. This 30 day challenge is intended to strengthen your habitual thinking in hopes of loving yourself—loving yourself void of anyone else's opinions about you. The less you focus on others, the less you'll worry how you fair in comparison to their online journey. Even if you're someone who is great at deciphering real life from online narratives, we still digest it in our subconsciousness. This is not an anti-social media campaign. It's a refocusing tool. This is not to encourage you to leave it forever. There are so many benefits. But your need to fall in love with yourself cannot happen when looking at everyone else.

You will remove pressure (real or not) to share and meet mommy standards (i.e. the snapback).

The less you share online, the less you worry about people's reactions and opinions on what you do. The less time you spend online during your postpartum healing, the less you'll feel pressured to show your "snap back". It's irrelevant and again, it's not real. Your body will do what it needs to do, on your own time. No matter how strong willed we believe we are, the more you look at everyone else, the more your subconscious digests who and what you're supposed to be. Removing these pressures will help you focus on who you were created to be—not who you'll morph into by following someone else. This will also alleviate the space for unsolicited advice and negativity. And force you to find inspiration from within.

You will have more energy to parent.

Social media is a social experiment that was designed to play on people's most vulnerable areas of the psyche. It was created to get us addicted. So taking a break during this time can help you re-prioritize where you put what little energy you have left. The more energy you have to parent, the better you'll feel. The better you feel, the better baby feels. 30 days isn't a long time, but if you're addicted it will be extremely hard to shake it. The great news is that you're worth more than any addiction. Empowering your mind is worth missing out on posts. You're worth it.

You will feel renewed.

With each day that you write what you love about yourself, you will in fact start to love those things. Even if it is made up, your brain won't know the difference. Taking the time away from social media will retrain your brain into receiving feedback loops from the smiles and laughs of your baby, versus the likes from friends and strangers online. The more you feel validated, the more energy you'll exert into replicating the action. Essentially, the more we feel validated by our babies, the more we will focus on them and not the reactions of others on how we parent them.

During your 30 day challenge to loving yourself, you'll finally find moments of stillness you didn't think existed. You'll find moments of complete silence — which scares may people because it ignites self-reflection (the start of humbly being honest with ourselves). These 30 days will help to focus and then re-focus you. It will help to put things in a more renewed perspective. It will allow you the time to just be and to wallow in all of the blessings you have. Doing this during the postpartum phase will be a great way to help empower yourself, combat baby blues or postpartum depression, and may be much more feasible before your baby starts walking around.

It will cause you to be present, which is essential because this time is nothing but a quick moment. It will pass and it's crucial we don't spend it on our phones or in a state of perpetually powerless thoughts. Cherish this moment and start to love yourself right now where you are. Challenge yourself to do something you've never done, because it's the only way to get what you've never had. You must do something different and refuting negative thoughts about yourself is the first step. You'll be amazed at how many negative things we say to ourselves daily. It serves no purpose and it shows a lack of gratefulness to the very powers that created us. Through humility, by releasing fears and insecurities, by choosing to love ourselves, we will rewire our brains and those vision boards will be a foreshadowing of all that is to come for you and your family. Keep going. You got this!

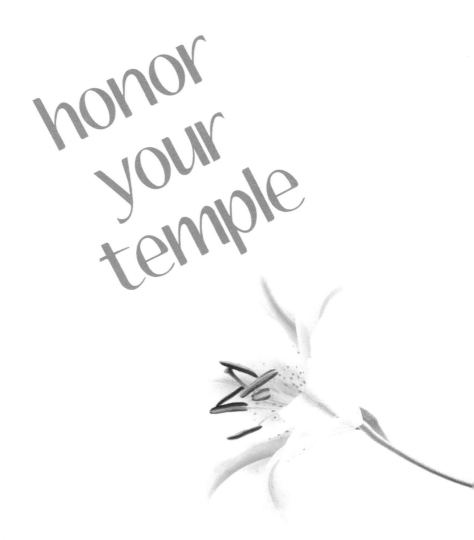

honor your temple

chapter 20

Sacrifice: Learning How and When to Let Go

With a renewed perspective, you can find joy in your evolving sense of freedom. Your fresh identity does not take away from the things you loved before motherhood (hobbies, hopes, dreams, et cetera). Motherhood simply elevates them. When we cannot do everything we desire in the exact moment we wish to do them, like in the past, it tends to magnify the things that "made" us who we were. Fortunately, we define who we are and how we grow based on the thoughts we possess in our minds. Now isn't the time to give up on your happiness — rather, it's simply time to prioritize.

Parenting is exhausting. Hence, why it's so important to channel your energy into things that truly require your attention, as not to burn yourself out dealing with things that hold no merit and add zero value to your newly evolved self. The truth is, there isn't a lot of extra time or energy to spare. Spending energy chasing an old way of life is exhausting and pointless. The old ways aren't coming back and the beauty is that this new journey is worth letting it go and moving forward. The past is behind you. Now is the time to enjoy discovering (or rediscovering) your newly evolving passions.

During this process, it's also essential to allow yourself time to find your new rhythm and routine. It likely won't happen overnight. The more patient you can be with yourself and the more you acknowledge the incredible job you're doing (because we definitely don't do it enough, if ever), the less stressful the transition can be. The more you allow yourself time to learn your new role, the more you can find peace and excitement for the future.

It's also important to retrain your love and expectancy of time. Things that once took you 30 minutes may now take you four days. For example, laundry that normally took an hour, may drag on for two weeks. Whereby it could normally take me about six months to write the *Hello, Hello: The Inspirational Guide to Motherhood* series, it actually took me two years. I would write while nursing, whenever the babies were napping, when the babies were playing together and sometimes in between each bite of food I would give them. At 15 months apart, there is never any real down time. And in those moment of complete silence and stillness, I was ready to sleep.

Overtime, the crazy ways I would attempt to just get a sentence or two out became a bit comical — but that was because I allowed myself to be okay with however long the process took. I knew my dream and I knew my priorities — to help you. I knew how quickly I wanted to get the books out as a means to help so many moms, but the truth was that with two babies under two, I just didn't have the luxury of time as I did before. I would write whenever I could and if there were times when I was just too tired (or when my family required 100% of my time), then I would focus on the tasks at hand and get back to writing when I was capable. That ranged from one day to a full month at times. I could have been frustrated with the process, but it was all about the perspective. There were absolutely days where I would be in the middle of a sentence, only to have to quickly change a poop diaper and then be completely out of my writing swing. Though it took longer than anticipated, I finished. You must allow yourself the space to go with the flow and not put unnecessary pressures on your dreams. What is meant for you will be — as long as you know without a slither of doubt that they will be so. You'll get there. Give it time.

While things may take longer to get done, remember this is just a season. Soon enough, the babies will either be old enough to engage in more independent activity and/or have a schedule that is much more predictable. Your time of more freedom will come — it just may not be right away. And that is okay. In your newly revived sense of priorities, you still don't have to choose between career or your family. You can have both with a bit of creativity, patience and unshakable faith — but it will be unique to your situation. As you grow into your new role as mom, things will begin to fall into place as you allow it. Remember, you must simply focus on what you want exclusively. You cannot focus on what you fear, what you don't want, or what you wish was different. Those thoughts perpetuate a cycle of remaining where you are. Whatever you focus on will come to fruition.

By focusing exclusively on what you want, the energy is solely into the dream(s). This will relieve your mind and spirit of resentment of the things you cannot do as freely and enable you to find inspiration in your new space. By focusing on what you want and not worrying about how it will happen, you allow yourself the freedom to simply dream and work on your own terms. As long as you believe it and put in the work, it will happen — and the manner by which things just fall in your lap will astound you. *Remember: You have to do what you've never done, to get what you've never had.*

It's all about perspective. So here's a fresh perspective from me to you: ***Pregnancy is designed to strip away the old you (hence, why it can be so uncomfortable, painful and even miserable). It is the stripping away of all that you once were. Bringing forth life is the moment that ignites all that you are capable of becoming. And motherhood is the one thing that fills you up with all you are, all you were created to be and all you were destined to accomplish.***

Find gratefulness in the struggle. It may take more time than anticipated to get in the groove, but be patient with yourself and baby. Focus on your dreams and your goals and find joy in your journey. Motherhood is a blessing and is a helpmeet to your dreams (not the ending point or the deterrent). The more we can humble ourselves and quiet our ego, the less stressed we will find ourselves. Just breathe and allow time to move at your pace for your peace.

you are a goddess

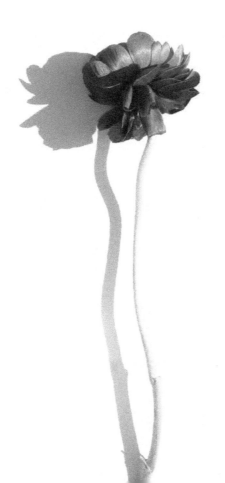

chapter 21

Hormonal Changes

*T*he shifts to our hormone levels post-delivery are extreme. Hence, why we tend to feel so out of whack as our body attempts to adjust to life post pregnancy, begins producing milk, increases prolactin, decreases estrogen, et cetera. During pregnancy, our levels of progesterone and estrogen are at all-time highs (possibly bettering your mood — save for those instances where pregnancy is rough). Post-delivery, the moment the placenta is pushed or taken out, there is a huge drop in our progesterone levels. For many who study the effects of hormonal changes post-delivery, it's thought to be one of the largest drops of hormones at one time for any human being at any point in their lifetime — that's huge!

The significant drop in our progesterone levels (the feel-good hormone) may be one culprit influencing your **baby blues** (defined as mood swings post-delivery). This imbalance between significantly low progesterone and higher levels of estrogen can also lead to decreased energy levels, cramping sensations (or irregular menstrual cycles), and mood swings (cue the irritability).

This drastic shift in your hormones play a huge role in how you feel during the 4th trimester. Hormones coupled with your lack of sleep, nerves, adjusting to your new responsibilities, not feeling understood, having unrealistic expectations (i.e. losing your stomach right after the baby comes out), judgment from others, stress — truly the list goes on and on — makes way for an emotional rollercoaster. You can easily and quickly feel like you're drowning in an ocean of your life, with no help in sight.

Other things such as self-perception can impact hormone levels as well. For example: When we stress over our bodies, this often leads to an obsession (whether conscious or subconscious). This can then impact our fatigue levels — being that our bodies are not designed to handle those levels of stress (nor that consistency). This increased level of fatigue then increases our cortisol levels. The increase in cortisol:

- makes your body store excess weight by holding on to fat
- and makes us crave more sugar and carbs—which then makes us more tired[9]

The importance of our thoughts should never be lost on us during this time (or for the rest of our lives for that matter). Our thoughts can directly contribute to hormones that are released in our bodies, making this introduction or reintroduction into motherhood much more physically and mentally taxing.

Another moment during this journey where we experience large shifts in our hormones is post breastfeeding, as you learned in the *Weaning* section of the *Breastfeeding* chapter. Weaning could occur anywhere from six weeks, well into baby's toddler years. Thus, the hormonal impact of motherhood does not simply go away after the six week timeline we are forced to give ourselves. Whereby most of us are cleared to continue on with life as if nothing happened around the 6-8 week mark, there is nothing normal going on. Realistically, it can take up to a full year for our bodies to fully heal from delivery — vaginal or via surgery. Everything in this first year is a part of a massive learning curve and it takes much longer than six weeks to find a rhythm that helps you feel somewhat normal again.

The truth is that postpartum care should be viewed with a much larger and longer lens. Even if you were to "feel" normal around six weeks (which is very likely), there is still much more healing your body and mind will go through. **We should truly look at postpartum care for the first year of our baby's life.** If we offer ourselves more time, we will place less pressure on ourselves to reach milestones of perfection.

The need to illustrate that we are fine, as if we didn't just produce life, is unhealthy and dangerous to our overall well-being. At six weeks and sometimes for the entire first year, our hormones are gravely unbalanced (all while our internal organs are shifting back into place and our bodies are adjusting to life on three hours of sleep each night). There truly is no need to act as if nothing major just happened. This just so happens to be the most major thing that could have happened. So we should treat it as such.

Baby milestones can go something like this:

- 1-2 months = colicky phase
- 3 months = adjusting to a schedule
- 5 months = laughing
- 6 months = trying solid food
- 7 months = teething
- 9 months = crawling
- 11—15 months = walking
- and so forth (obviously these vary drastically)

The point to be illustrated here is that, essentially every month there is a new milestone. The moment you "master" one thing, something else comes up as if right on cue (i.e. sleep regression). Adjusting to baby while also trying to reclaim your newly evolved self takes time. We must allow ourselves the time we need on a more holistic level. Rather than focusing on just the external appearance that we have it all together, we should truly allow ourselves the time to try and get things together in a manner that will really serve us in an empowered way. For some that may take three months (I haven't met this mom yet, but anything is possible — it could be you!), it may take 9 months, or even two years. Whatever the case, if we offer ourselves the proper time and space to heal and evolve, the less pressure we will place on ourselves (and the more likely we won't cause an increase in hormones that make the healing process harder — like that increased cortisol that encourages us to keep eating those doughnuts — ugh).

Our holistic being simply needs more time to heal. We should go into motherhood knowing that it will be hard, but with time and patience we will overcome the obstacles (which are really blessings to help us develop stronger character traits). Providing yourself that time to heal and expecting for it to be a journey until we find our rhythm, will help to alleviate unnecessary expectations and stress.

Simply put: give yourself time. There is no rush for anything. Don't compare your journey to anyone else's. We're all just figuring this thing out as we go. You have a lifetime to figure it out. There is no rush. Just breathe and let it be.

chapter 22

Postpartum Depression + Postpartum PTSD

ccording to the National Institute of Mental Health, **postpartum depression** is defined as:

> "...a mood disorder that can affect women after childbirth...leading to feelings of extreme sadness, anxiety and exhaustion that may make it difficult for them to complete daily care activities for themselves or for others."[10]

With much information written about postpartum depression, there is a still a huge misconception when it hits you, that it's somehow the equivalent to you being a bad mom — or that you were the cause of it. There are many things that impact postpartum depression in moms. Stress levels, sleep deprivation and hormonal changes are but a few things that increase the likelihood of developing levels of postpartum depression.

It's also important to give credit to how strong of a shift motherhood has on the wiring (and now re-wiring) or our brains. There are significant cognitive changes to our brains that most of us are completely unaware of on a conscious level. From pregnancy and beyond, our brains evolve to adapt to motherhood. Remember how the sense of smell was intensified during pregnancy? This is the brain's method of making us more apt to identifying potential dangers to our unborn baby via our sense of smell.

Post-delivery, our brain intensifies its level of validation and rewards circuits. Studies done on moms brains postpartum have illustrated the extreme sensitivity that develops in reaction to their babies. There is now a significant increase in emotional response to our baby (hence, why it can be heartbreaking to hear our baby crying rather than initially being angry or annoyed). The increase in reward circuits helps to regulate distress that moms would certainly experience without some sort of cognitive balancing act that aids our action—and allows us not to completely give up on motherhood after our baby has cried for an hour straight.

Another change to our brains includes an increased level of anxiety. This can absolutely contribute to depression, as moms are constantly worried about being inadequate or incapable of fully protecting our babies (fear). It's noted that these changes to our brains are intensified within the first few years of our children's life (which makes sense as it's typically the time where they're most susceptible to falls, bumps, bruises, eating the wrong things, et cetera).

The purpose of understanding how our intense levels of parenting are related to our brains and not just deciding to be overly protective, is to stress the importance of being honest about your feelings and asking for help. Whereby moms of older children might have a hard time remembering the exact ins and outs of what they did when their babies were young (it's also a much different time to parent in then it was just 10 years ago), finding moms who are going through what you are and have babies around the same age will be your saving grace. Trust me, we're all going through the same thing!

The less support you have as a mom, the higher likely your stress levels and the less likely you're to be able to identify and make changes to mitigate your postpartum depression. The capability of developing this form of depression is not contingent upon the amount of money you have, or even at times, the level of emotional support you have. But the more help you can find, the stronger your ability to beat it.

It's important to acknowledge that many of our woes as moms in the beginning of our journey connects with our feelings of being misunderstood, judged, unloved and alone or isolated from the world that was once our playground. There are times when a mom feels perfectly fine, until it's time to nurse. The mere act of breastfeeding can lead a mom to feeling extreme levels of loneliness. Having someone to communicate this to, who can truly empathize your situation (not merely intellectualize it — the difference between talking to someone with and without children) and who doesn't judge your feelings, will be essential in your journey to overcoming your postpartum depression — even if it is mild.

One study in particular by researchers at Baylor University has always stood out to me as I was doing my research for this book. It exemplified that, of all industrialized countries, the United States is not only the least safe place to have a baby (highest maternal death rate), but it also has the largest gap of happiness between parents and non-parents.[11] Essentially, these studies express that people are no longer finding the benefits of having children worth the happiness and joy that they give up. Part of this is due to the lack of programs offering education and help for moms, poor maternity and paternity leave options for working parents and poor vacation days — versus that of every other industrialized country. Basically, it feels too expensive and much harder than it is beneficial.

Being that significant changes to these areas which could positively and powerfully impact mothers won't happen with the archaic patriarchal view of the needs of women still in power, the change will have to happen with us. We have to find a community whereby communication is not only encouraged, but is the norm. You must find your safe space—and this may or may not be online. With the advent of social media, there are lots of instances where we feel connected to others, but are completely missing out on the power of personal interactions. Sometimes the act of just physically being around other moms can have a wonderful impact on your psyche. Just the simple notion of going outside to get some fresh air can completely change your mood—instantly.

Even if we do all of the things deemed necessary, it's still possible to develop some form of postpartum depression. Missing out on our past child free life is a sure way to develop it —which is something many moms experience. This does not make you a bad mom in any way—it makes you human. Experiencing feelings of regret, confusion, even irritation can happen and it happens to more women than what's reported (being as though many women either don't share that they have it, or may not know they have it). It isn't the fact we have these thoughts, but rather the manner in which we can identify them and redirect our thinking to a more empowered space.

It has often been reported that approximately 50% of moms experience the baby blues, with approximately 20% experiencing postpartum depression and about 1% experiencing postpartum psychosis. The likelihood that this is gravely under-reported is highly plausible; hence, the importance of guarding ourselves with as much information as we can in hopes of helping ourselves and others.

The feelings of baby blues or postpartum depression often come with a lot of doubt, at times self-hatred and many regrets. It can be hard—almost impossible—for moms to find a safe space to share their true feelings without being judged or made to feel ashamed about those feelings. Having the baby blues does not make you ungrateful and the more we can offer compassion to ourselves and others during this time, the more of an impact we can make towards true healing for mothers around the globe. Compassion is key.

It's important to be honest about your feelings, as this is a large component to strengthening your resolve to find healing. Remember, you're not a terrible mother should you find yourself dealing with postpartum depression. As natural a phenomenon as motherhood is, is it not always instinctual! There is a lot to learn about being a mom that seems like it would just come naturally. There are certainly some things that do, but through our humility we can accept that there are lots of components that just aren't as instinctual as we would like to believe. It's okay to be confused, feel regret, confusion, et cetera. It's merely about how we address and overcome.

Though postpartum depression is starting to gain more traction in mainstream conversations, postpartum PTSD often times goes overlooked. While postpartum depression is a result of hormonal changes, **postpartum post-traumatic stress syndrome** is a result of trauma (or perceived trauma) during the delivery process. Studies have shown approximately 9% of moms have experienced postpartum PTSD (and these are just the numbers reported). Psychologist Susanne Babbel of Psychology Today notes that some causes of this form of PTSD include[12]:

- premature birth
- still birth or loss of baby post successful delivery
- having a baby in NICU
- prolapsed cord during delivery
- extreme difficulties during pregnancy, labor and or delivery (i.e. unplanned hysterectomy, hemorrhage, severe tears, et cetera)
- unplanned cesarean section
- use of vacuum or forceps
- women with a history of sexual abuse and/or trauma

Author Sharon Praissman Fisher suggests that "feelings of powerlessness, poor communication, and/or lack of support and reassurance during the delivery can also contribute to postpartum PTSD."[13]

While there may seem to be a bit of hopelessness in developing either case, the great news is that they're both treatable. Moms who develop post-traumatic stress syndrome should absolutely seek professional help to aid in the healing process—in hopes to avoid the development of the most severe cases. If you develop PTSD, it's essential you treat yourself with the compassion your heart desires. Neither postpartum depression or post-traumatic stress syndrome are minimal instances; nor something that should be swept under the rug by anyone—including your physician.

Many times, moms find healing via open commutation. Talking it out can lead to finding other moms who are or have been exactly where you are. As you find healing, you'll then become the light in a dark place for other moms struggling as well. By helping others, you'll start to find strength in your own journey and recognize again just how powerful you are. Remember to plant seeds in your mind that will produce fruit not poison. Honesty, self-care and compassion can be the start to nurturing the healing you need. Never give up. You'll make it through and you'll find happiness again. You will. And there are many moms out there who can attest to that very thing you can't seem to shake. This book is a testament to the fact that you can and you'll make it through, as did I. Keep going mama! Joy is right around the corner. And the more you laugh, even if it's fake, the more you put yourself on the right track!

chapter 23

Your Support System

One of the key ingredients to developing postpartum depression is feeling alone, isolated and overwhelmed. Many times, a lack of support can be a huge contributing factor. Regardless of what you have heard, how strong you are, or your thoughts on how you'll be different once you have a baby, the truth is simple: **we all need help**.

You must find your community of support because there will always come a day when you must lean on them to get you through—to make you feel normal, to ensure you that it's going to be okay and to let you know that you aren't alone. Never be afraid or ashamed to ask for help. Find people you trust and who love you through and through. You'll be your most vulnerable and will need people who can put their own feelings aside to aid you no matter what.

Establishing your support system is important and shouldn't be taken lightly. Being friends with someone for a long time, for example, doesn't automatically ensure they will be able to provide the support you need in this specific and precious time. Just because someone is family also does not mean they're who you need around you during your most vulnerable moments. Some key components you'll need for your support system include, but are not limited to:

- non-judgmental (they should never tell you to just "get over it" unless that is the type of support you require)
- sensitive to your healing, needs and emotional vulnerability
- can physically help with the baby (so you can get a real break and not have to entertain)
- is encouraging and understanding
- is a great listener
- checks on you even when you don't ask
- has a calm, peaceful and drama/stress free aura (if they're stressed, it will undoubtedly make you stressed)

For some, you may already have that person (or the group of people) who immediately come to mind. This might be an easy feat for you and if so, take advantage of how incredibly blessed you are. For those who may need some time to really find your support system, a great help is to establish that support system prior to delivery. Once baby is here, you'll rarely have the time to think about anything other than baby and sleep.

It's important for you to have help that can fulfill essential needs—not someone you have to exert energy into entertaining or teaching how to help (yet, if you have the time and patience to do so, then do it—that too is awesome!). You'll likely need someone(s) who can help with laundry, food, giving you time to nap and maybe some nighttime feedings. These things will start to fall into your routine as baby adjusts to life outside of the womb, so don't worry—you won't need the help in this particular manner forever. This is just crucial for the early weeks/months as you heal and navigate your way through the start of this journey.

It's also important to remember to cut yourself some slack. You don't have to be and do all things at all times. Sometimes chores will get put on the back burner. Decide what truly needs to get done to protect your sanity. For everything else, allow your support system to help—or just do it another day. It's okay. If there are things you cannot live without (i.e. a messy kitchen before bed), then sacrifice the laundry one night to clean the kitchen. Over time your routine with baby will help you establish your needs and desires within the schedule. Cleanliness is important, but it will come over time. It's true that the more organized things are in your physical space, the less chaotic your mind feels. But in the beginning of your 4th trimester, cut yourself some slack. Do what you need, relinquish what can wait and don't judge it.

Don't try to fit everything in. Strive for peace not perfection. I personally could not ever go to bed before the baby's toys and books were put away. In the beginning it felt like a chore, but I knew when I woke up to a clean house the next morning I would calm and at peace (even if for a short stint). The more at peace I was, the more calm and at peace my babies were. Over time, cleaning up before bed became a part of my routine with the babies. Now, every night before getting ready for bed, we all clean up our books and toys together before heading to take a bath.

As simple as it sounds, it has always been a huge part of my sanity. The less chaotic the house, the more normal I felt. A friend of mine, on the other hand, couldn't fathom the thought of putting anything away. Once the babies were down, she didn't want to even think about a baby toy or book. It was her time and she owned it. That was her peace and her peace made her babies at peace. The point is to follow your gut, listen to your heart, do what you need to do and ask for help when and where you need it. In time you'll find your rhythm and you'll start to find your independence again.

chapter 24

Vitamins + Healthy Eating

*A*nother contributing factor of postpartum depression comes from our lack of energy and sleep; hence, why it's so important to get out of the house when you can and get some sunlight. The natural vitamin D your body will receive will rejuvenate you mentally and physically and can give you energy (especially if you go for a walk). The foods we eat are also essential to our overall well-being postpartum—which can be extremely hard to focus on when all of our attention is on baby and the sleep we miss.

If and when the time comes that your body feels depleted, vitamins can be of great assistance (especially if taking them from the start of your postpartum journey). Certain vitamins are known to help replenish your body during the healing process and can aid in areas that are being stripped away due to breastfeeding (i.e. calcium).

Taking vitamins post-delivery is completely optional, of course and depends on your body. With a bit of research, you can find brands that suit you. Some of the best vitamins for your body during the 4th trimester include, but are not limited to:

- **Postnatal Vitamin:** there are vitamins tailored for postpartum care, inclusive of nursing moms as well (the goal is to help replenish your body with the extra nutrients it needs)

- **Calcium Magnesium:** if you are not getting enough nutrients, your body will pull calcium from your bones in order to produce your milk — your cal/mag vitamin will help to nourish your body, strengthen your bones and help balance your digestive tract — they can be taken together or separately, as magnesium is a great vitamin to aid with relaxation and sleep

- **Vitamin D:** this is important for baby (which they get from your breastmilk in the first six months) and is often added as an oral dosage around the six month mark to avoid deficiencies — this should be added to your regiment as well as most new moms experience an iron deficiency during pregnancy and 4th trimester

- **Vitamins B and C:** help with immunity and energy (which is extremely beneficial since your body is more susceptible to sickness with little to no sleep) — breastfeeding alone isn't the culprit of your constant sickness postpartum, but rather it's your depleted nutrients and exhaustion that is lowering your body's ability to fight off infection

- **Probiotics:** important to help promote and maintain a healthy gut

Remember that your body is going through a major transition. A healthy, well rounded nutrition plan is best—and establishing a plan is probably your best bet to making sound choices rather than grabbing quick snacks. While some may have this down to a science, most moms (like myself) struggle with finding balance between taking care of the baby(s) and properly feeding ourselves. It felt so time consuming for me to focus on the proper meals and I never felt like I had any down time to enjoy my food anyway — especially since I stood up during each meal and ate so fast like I was in a food eating contest. For those who struggle as I did, trying to choose healthier snacks can be beneficial to establishing better eating habits.

Doing your best is all you should strive for in this moment. Don't beat yourself up if your diet isn't perfect (which it probably isn't unless you're a dietician, a cook, someone who really loves the topic of nutrition, or have your own personal chef). Wherever you fall on the spectrum, just remember to prioritize your energy. Maybe one week your focus is solely on sleep training — the next week, finding a baby sitter — the next week, teething, et cetera. When nutrition becomes the goal for the week, then focus on just that and allow yourself time to refocus and establish your healthier goals. Don't strive for perfection, strive for peace of mind. Do what you can, when you can. Preparation will always be key in eating healthier — but sometimes life just gets the best of us. With patience and persistence, you'll find the balance your eating habits need. In the meantime, take your vitamins to help supplement possible deficiencies. They will be key in helping you get back on your feet.

Remember to listen to your body and refuel when you need. Eat small meals often (like you did during pregnancy) to help avoid nausea, light headedness, or becoming so hungry that you rely of whatever you can get your hands on (which always seems to be the chips or cookies). Everything is a season and this moment is one as well. You won't always have to eat standing up and you won't always feel like finding nutritional wholeness is a challenge. It will get easier, especially if you have made it up in your mind that it will be so.

Simply try and make the best of each day by being your best. Take it day by day (and take your vitamins every day). Also keep in mind that no matter how many vitamins you take and no matter how many vegetables you eat, the more stress you harbor, the more your body will take away blood from your digestive tract and internal organs and push more blood to your extremities. Even when doing the best we can health wise, stress can make it null and void. Find what works for you. Take some time to just breathe and find the things you're thankful for. It will get hard and that is okay. No judgment. No guilt. You got this!

chapter 25

Baby Sleep (Tummy or Back)

F iguring out our babies sleeping patterns and preferences is also a season (though often feeling like a never ending one — trust me, you'll make it through this as well). There is much information focused on the importance of sleep for our babies, as well as methods to aid their sleeping journeys. Each baby is different and the most effective strategy for baby may differ from other moms you know. Educating yourself is ultimately the best strategy — as there is tons of information and many resources to help offer suggestions and tips for your set of circumstances. One of the biggest questions we often ask ourselves, aside from how much sleep they need, is how they should sleep: tummy or back?

In 1992, the American Academy of Pediatrics (AAP) changed the recommendation for babies to start sleeping on their backs versus their stomachs as a means to reduce the likelihood of developing SIDS (sudden infant death syndrome). Since that time, the numbers have shown a drastic decrease in the SIDS death rates. Though the numbers may be compelling, as a parent it can still be a difficult decision to make — especially when baby prefers sleeping on their tummy (and sleeps better at that).

Plagiocephaly (aka Flathead Syndrome)

The one thing you should remind yourself when making this decision is that, it's a personal one and completely up to you. While research has shown a drop in the SIDS rates, there is still a misconception about the manner by which babies should sleep and lay on their backs. While the proposed benefits of placing babies on their backs may be enough to make you choose this option, it's essential to monitor the length of time baby is on their back to help prevent flathead syndrome—which has drastically increased since the change came about from the AAP.

Flathead syndrome, also known as plagiocephaly, is the flattening of the skull due to too much pressure on the areas of soft tissue. The more babies sleep, play and nap on their backs, the more they press on the soft tissue on the backs of their skulls, causing it to flatten their heads (remember the importance of tummy time!). Fortunately, flathead syndrome is treatable. If minor, you may simply need to decrease the amount of back time and introduce more tummy time. For more severe cases, cranial orthotic therapy (the use of a molding helmet), may be necessary to restructure the soft tissue.

If placing baby on their back works for you, do it—but remember to balance it out with sufficient tummy time. If, on the other hand, baby prefers sleeping on their tummy and is able to lift and move their head (to avoid suffocating), then you should listen to your mommy gut before anything else. There are other ways to help reduce the chances of baby having SIDS, if sleeping on the back doesn't work. If this is the case for you, don't stress — you're not alone. Many parents allow their babies to sleep on their tummy if it's most effective for sleeping. In some instances, a baby may roll from their backs to belly very early on (as did both of my babies). If that's the case and they're sleeping well, leave them. If they're strong enough to hold their head up and roll over, they won't suffocate. There are cases when a baby may suffer from gas, acid reflux, or other digestive troubles that make sleeping on the tummy therapeutic. If that's the case, they're sleeping well and you feel good about your choice to allow them to sleep that way, then do it.

SIDS

The purpose is not to convince you to disregard the research from the AAP. The goal is simply to encourage you to follow your gut and do what's best for you and baby. It's also important not to stress or beat yourself up if you have to deviate from what is suggested. At the end of the day, every baby is different and placing a baby on their back or tummy to ensure the safest and most effective sleeping habits is a personal choice. If you're interested in other ways by which to **decrease the risk of SIDS**, the following list offers some tips (void of monitors placed on babies — as they don't reduce the risks of SIDS, but rather can increase anxiety levels in parents):

- **Remove anything that could cause choking or suffocation hazards in the crib (no toys or soft bedding).** For the first year or so, baby won't need a pillow or fluffy blankets. This is particularly important for the first couple of months as it could pose as a risk for suffocation or smothering. Rather than placing blankets on baby, find warmer zip up onesies that can cover their hands and feet instead.

- **Keep baby cool (monitor overheating).** Overheating has been found to contribute to SIDS. If you discover baby is starting to overheat, don't panic. If you're nursing, give baby breastmilk—as it will help to normalize their temperate. Offer baby a lukewarm bath (not cold)—sponge bath is also applicable—or wipe them down with a cool cloth. In time, you'll find the best temperature for baby's room. Some like it cooler or warmer—often times depending on the manner by which you sleep (baby will likely adjust according to your habits).

- **Keep smoke away from baby.** Not only should you avoid smoking, but avoid being around smoke. According to Webmd, *"Babies born to women who smoked during pregnancy die from SIDS three times more often than babies born to nonsmokers."*[14] The same applies post-delivery if baby is simply around smoke.

- **Keep baby in your room (proceed with extreme caution if baby is in the same bed).** Keeping baby in the room with you for at least the first six months or so has shown to decrease the likelihood of developing SIDS. Previously called "crib death", it was thought that babies who were left alone in a separate room stopped breathing because they did not hear the breath of their mothers at night. Transitioning baby to their own room is an exciting time for parents to get back to normal, but there is truly no rush. If you decide to co-sleep, be cautious about suffocation dangers—including your own breast. Nursing at night can be extremely exhausting. There will be times when you wake up to find baby sleep on your nipple (it happens). Being careful, particularly in the early days when your breasts are abnormally full, is essential to preventing suffocation. Also, be very cautious that neither you nor your spouse rolls over onto baby if they're in the bed with you.

- **Breastfeed if you can.** Studies have shown breastfeeding decreases the risks of SIDS by upwards of 50%. Just another incredible benefit of nursing.

- **Never give honey to your baby.** Honey is a food whereby bacteria causes toxins to be released in baby's body, resulting in botulism (which can lead to breathing difficulties and the development of SIDS).

Remember that these are all tips medical professionals have studied and deemed effective in reducing the risks. Unfortunately, no one knows for sure what causes it. This is why it's so important to listen to your intuition—your mommy gut is your greatest asset (often times more than any google search or study). Try to avoid making decisions based on fear. Do the best you can and marvel at how beautiful baby grows and thrives.

chapter 26

Pelvic Weakness (Incontinence)

Pelvic incontinence refers to leakage due to laughing, sneezing, coughing, running, jumping or lifting. During the often referenced timeline of 6-8 weeks healing time, you'll surely experience incontinence. The kegels you have been doing since pregnancy will be a great help during this time, as your pelvic floor beings to regain its strength (as noted in *Hello, Hello: The Inspirational Guide to Pregnancy*). Allowing yourself time to heal properly (i.e. refraining from working out until you're medically cleared), will aid in strengthening your pelvic floor—and even encourage your body to end up stronger than it was before delivery.

Whether you're someone who hasn't done kegels before, or have done them and continue to experience incontinence well beyond the 8-week postpartum mark, there is nothing to fret.

Postpartum urinary incontinence is a common ailment many women experience. According to the site Baby Center:

> *Normally your nerves, ligaments and pelvic*
> *floor muscles work together to support your*
> *bladder and keep the urethra closed so urine*
> *doesn't leak. Over-stretching or injuring these*
> *during pregnancy or childbirth may cause*
> *urine leakage.*[15]

Though you're much more likely to develop incontinence post vaginal delivery, some women have been found to experience pelvic muscle weakness post-cesarean section as well. Optimal pushing positions during delivery can help to reduce the trauma and overexertion on your pelvic floor (as explained in the *Optimal Pushing Positions* chapter of *Hello, Hello: The Inspirational Guide to Pregnancy*). For example, pushing on all fours or while in a squat position allows gravity to aid in the delivery without having to push as much, compared to the intense strain caused by pushing on your back.

Other risks for incontinence include:

- gestational diabetes

- assisted vaginal delivery

- birthing a large baby or prolonged pushing (most times due to numbness from medication)

- having multiple vaginal deliveries

- smoking

If you battle with postpartum urinary incontinence, the great news is that with some work it can strengthen. Kegels will continue to be your best friend in terms of strengthening and tightening your pelvic floor. For those who are interested in other forms of pelvic exercises, practicing yoga may be another means to tap into your body and focus on holistically strengthening yourself. It's also important to remember your stool softeners, as extreme pushing can weaken the pelvic floor and make the incontinence worse (prolonging healing time).

Exercising prematurely, straining, or lifting heavy items (even your toddlers) too soon, can continuously weaken your pelvic floor. Though it's exciting to finally get back to moving the way you did before pregnancy, it's important to allow your body the time it needs to heal. Moving too soon can possibly make your incontinence worse.

In the end, don't stress. Wearing panty liners will be helpful in the meantime and with a little work and patience, your body will start to heal. Don't be ashamed and don't feel alone. You just had a baby — so allow time for your body to regain strength. You just overcame a huge feat, treat yourself as such. It'll get better. Just remember those kegels.

chapter 27

Diastisis Recti

Another major reason to avoid rushing to exercise prior to the six weeks healing time, is the development of **diastisis recti**. This occurs when the muscles in the abdomen separate and drastically move away from one another. During pregnancy, the hormone relaxin allows for this separation to happen without too much pain. But the manner by which it took 9 months to separate, is the manner by which it can take upwards of two months for the healing process (closure) to begin.

In most instances, the tissues that stretched in your abdomen will heal and being to tighten again on their own. Once the space between the upper and lower parts of your abdomen are small enough (whereby you cannot fit your fingers in between when pressing on it), it's typically a signal you can slowly begin your abdomen workouts. Starting an abdominal workout too soon can actually cause more strain on the tissue and create more space and damage. Time is truly your greatest asset during your postpartum healing.

There are also times when the healing process of the tissue just doesn't occur (which is noted for roughly 40% of moms). There are some instances which are more extreme than others. For example, a mom who has had multiple cesarean sections may have severe damage to the tissue, whereby they're able to essentially take their hand and feel the floor when pressing on their stomachs while laying on their back. While it can be extremely gut wrenching and discouraging, there are ways to promote healing of the abdomen.

One of the best ways to check if you have diastisis recti includes lying on your back with knees bent and lightly lifting your head upwards to contract your abdomen. Take your hand and feel the space between your abdomen. If by six months the gap hasn't closed, it's likely you have developed it. Sometimes lightly lifting your head from a laying position (only 10 times a day) can be enough to start promoting healing post-delivery. When healing doesn't occur, doing more abdominal work will make the problem worse. This will be the time to look into specialized postnatal diastisis therapy exercises.

Physical therapy is a great way to begin strengthening the damaged area. This will likely require someone who specializes in this particular diagnosis, as regular therapy won't work. If you plan to get pregnant again, it may be advisable to find healing prior to your next pregnancy. If you're done having babies, surgery may be an option as well. Fortunately, many women find healing with specialized techniques for core work or specialized physical therapy.

Though it can be emotionally taxing, it's important to remember you're not alone—with approximately three million women being diagnosed yearly. You can find healing, though it will take time. But as you now know, time is your best friend during this postpartum healing journey. Motherhood is never-ending, reinforcing the notion that rushing doesn't help with anything. Allowing yourself the necessary time to heal post-delivery will ultimately help reduce your overall healing time. If your body needs more attention and care, then allow yourself even more time. You can get back to the body you desire and the more you work and take care of yourself, the more likely you'll end up with the body you never really thought you could have: one you love unconditionally.

chapter 28

Recovering From
Cesarean Section

Recovery from vaginal delivery is different than that of recovery from major surgery. If you're so fortunate enough to be able to take the 6-8 weeks needed to heal, you should take advantage of the full amount of time. By waiting the 6-8 week period, you'll allow your body the ability to get stronger prior to the start of your workouts and your regular routine. Reminding yourself that working out (or doing any other inadvisable activities) too soon can actually cause more damage and prolong healing, will be essential during your postpartum journey. Even if you "feel" ready (which is extremely likely), your internal organs, ligaments, muscles and tissue still need the time.

In the United States, approximately 1/3 of babies are born via cesarean section. Even amidst the normalcy of such surgery, many women are still struggling to cope during the postpartum healing phase. Having your support system (who can physically be there with you), open communication about your emotional well-being and staying in-tune with your physical and psychological scars will be gravely important during this process.

First thing to keep in mind, which is lifesaving: **listen to your body**. You must demand that everyone take your feelings seriously (no matter what that constitutes). No one knows your body better than you and regardless of how many degrees a doctor has or how many births a nurse has attended, no single person will be able to be as in-tune with your physical needs than you. If you ever feel disregarded or brushed off by your medical staff, you and your support system should continuously press them until you have what you need — or consider changing providers.

As discussed in *Hello, Hello: The Inspirational Guide to Delivery*, unfortunate desensitization, traditional methodologies, forced medical intervention and institutionalized discriminatory practices (conscious or unconscious) have immensely contributed to the quantifiable data which shows that most maternal deaths and near death occurrences are in fact preventable. **It's imperative to always remember that you hold the power.** Though you should never have to fight for the right for your pain to be taken seriously, you may have to. And if you do, you and your support team must fight to be heard and taken care of as if your life depends on it — because it does.

While most of the attention post-delivery is on the baby, your needs as mom are just as vital. With major surgery comes increased chances of complications such as hemorrhage, placental retention, infection, high blood pressure, et cetera.

Missed vital signs or prolonged checkups (i.e. checking blood levels, blood pressure, ensuring there is no blood in the catheter, et cetera.), can lead to devastating results. By remaining vigilant and ensuring everyone around you is acutely aware of the fact that you need vital attention will be your greatest asset during your recovery.

The good news is that, as more attention is being placed on the need to better care for mothers postpartum, you'll more than likely be able to go home and safely start your healing journey there. There are a few things which are important to know—that (hopefully) can help the recovery process from your cesarean section feel more manageable and less of a shock to the system:

Expect nausea post-surgery.

Nausea from the medication can last upwards of 48 hours post-surgery. Other side effects may include itching or the shakes (another result of medication and narcotics wearing out of your system).

Breastfeeding may be challenging.

This may be the case, especially during the first couple of days. If you're unable to nurse baby immediately post-delivery, as is the case for a majority of moms after surgery, this may make it more challenging to establish an early rhythm with your little one (especially if they're offered a bottle with formula prior to nursing — but it's still possible to successfully breastfeed if this happens). Pain from the incision area, muscle soreness and the inability to move freely to your desired positions may also make it difficult. Laying on your side may help alleviate the pain. It's important to reach out to other moms who have experienced the same thing, to find effective and less painful ways to nurse your beautiful baby.

Things to know about your incision.

Every mom's surgical experience varies. For example, some women may actually feel the tugging and cutting sensations, while others are completely numb. Similarly, incision recoveries vary as well. One benefit of the United States finally adopting the German method of using the low transverse cut, is that incision scars are much smaller and less visible then in the past (by your bikini line). Post surgery, you'll either have your staples removed, or simply let your dissolvable sutures heal on their own.

It's important to leave the incision alone (especially in the first week) as it begins to close and heal. For the first two weeks, you won't be able to lift anything heavy — including your other children. You'll also have to skip your bath or swimming pool during this time as well. It's important to ensure that your incision is puffy and pink. If it bleeds or oozes, turns red, or if you have a spike in temperature, this could suggest a possible infection.

After your six-week checkup, the incision will be considered "healed", though it may maintain its bruised color for the next few months. There are also some moms whose incision **keloids** (raised scar tissue post healing). Some doctors might suggest an injection of steroids into the incision to help reduced the raised scar tissue (a personal decision — be sure to do your research). There is also a chance of persistent itching or slight to permanent numbness.

The beauty of your incision is that it's indeed your battle scar. Whenever you look in the mirror, you'll have a beautiful reminder of just how much of a fight your body endured to bring forth your heartbeat made manifest. It's a constant window into your soul — showcasing just how far you were willing to go to save your baby. It's magnanimous and so are you.

You will have postpartum bleeding.

Though it may not be as much as those with vaginal delivery, your uterus must still contract in order to reduce to its normal size and prevent hemorrhage. This may result in nurses cleaning your vaginal area multiple times post-delivery to ensure that it stays clean and begins healing properly. Bleeding can last up to six weeks and will subside over time.

Keep a soft pillow nearby for the first few weeks.

Laughing, coughing and sneezing may be painful post-surgery. Having something soft to apply light pressure on the area may be helpful in relieving some discomfort. Waist supports (similar to those used during pregnancy) offer a stabilizing effect to your abdominal area. The support may be extremely beneficial as your organs shift back in place, your abdominal wall begins to strengthen and your core begins the healing process.

Walk when you can.

You've probably heard moms say how walking and moving around post-surgery was one of the best things to initiate the physical and mental healing process. Don't feel confined to your bed. The less you move, the worse you're likely to feel. Remember to take your time and move at your own pace. Getting out of bed for the first couple of weeks can vary from uncomfortable to excruciating. But, staying in bed is counterproductive to your healing. When you can, if you can, will yourself to move — ensuring that it's within the boundaries of aiding your healing rather than overdoing or overexerting yourself (which would add time to the overall healing process).

Remember your stool softeners.

During pregnancy, relaxin caused things to stretch and slow down — including your digestive tract. Post-delivery, it takes some time for your gut to normalize. It's imperative not to strain to use the restroom (as this could increase your chances of developing urinary incontinence). If you're breastfeeding, you don't want to take laxatives because you won't want to flush your system of all of the good nutrients your body needs for milk production (it also could give baby a severe bout of diarrhea). A combination of your realigning intestinal tract, pain medications, lack of sleep and a change in your diet could also contribute to digestive complications (most notably constipation). Stool softeners (and probiotics) can help mitigate the fear and discomfort of bowel movements. Adding this to your daily routine, along with simple exercises (i.e. walking) should really help to get things moving again.

You may experience postpartum edema (water retention).

Many moms experience intense swelling post-surgery. This is caused by increased levels of fluid in the body (including fluids given through your IV) that haven't flushed out of your body. The goal is to increase circulation to get things flowing. Tips to help reduce swelling and increase circulation include:

- walking
- compression socks/leggings
- drinking water (lemon water helps to reduce inflammation)
- using cabbage leaves (especially for engorged breasts) as its anti-inflammatory properties help to draw out fluids from the body
- prop your feet up
- reduce caffeine intake and increase your potassium
- reduce your sodium intake (take salt out of your diet)
- avoid processed foods (harbors too much sugar)
- avoid standing or sitting for long periods of time (move your body)

- get a leg, hand, or arm massage to encourage circulation
- try acupuncture or chiropractic services to align your body and promote healing and circulation

It may take a few extra days for your body to flush out the extra fluids from your IV and medication. Try some of the tips above and remember that this is just a season. It will pass.

Healing your mind is as vital as your body.

The most important component that is often largely overlooked is the healing of psychological scar tissue. It's imperative not to judge your birth, regardless of anyone's opinions on how it turned out. Even if surgery was a surprise and completely opposite of your desires, the most important thing is that you and baby survived and are thriving. It does no good to judge or beat yourself up. Having brought forth life via cesarean section does not make you any less of a mom or a woman. We must drop the guilt. Never allow anyone (not even yourself) make you feel weak, unworthy, or as if you took the easy way out. You didn't. Surgery is no easy way. You're a superhero. You won the fight — and it was a life threatening fight. It may not have gone as planned, but the great news is you can still have the birth of your dreams in the future. Vaginal births after cesareans (VBAC) are possible and your hopes are not lost (as explained in detail in *The Truth About VBACs* chapter of *Hello, Hello: The Inspirational Guide to Delivery*). Stay empowered in your thoughts and continue to allow yourself time to heal on a holistic level (mind, body and spirit).

chapter 29

Postpartum Pre-Eclampsia

While many mothers are aware of preeclampsia during pregnancy, very few are aware of the rare condition that occurs up to six weeks postpartum. High blood pressure and high levels of protein in the urine (similar to preeclampsia), are signs of the condition post-delivery. While a mom can deliver a perfectly healthy baby, it's still possible to develop (though rare) after the baby is born — stressing the importance of following up with your doctor or midwife and paying close attention to your body.

Symptoms of postpartum preeclampsia are the same as those during pregnancy:

- severe headaches
- intense stomach pains

- vision changes (blurriness, short term blindness, et cetera)

- nausea and vomiting

- shortness of breath

Paying attention to your body post-delivery can be the key to saving your life. Knowing the warning signs may also be life-saving, as many doctors may attribute your feelings to sleep deprivation or the norms of having a newborn. If something feels off, trust your instincts! At 32 years young, a perfectly healthy mom of twins suddenly lost her vision at four weeks postpartum. After weeks of notifying her doctors of severe migraines, she suffered from a stroke — at 32. After a full year of recovery (including regaining her vision), she is finally starting to feel like herself again. It can truly happen to anyone. Stay vigilant, have your support system and never brush off how you're feeling or things you may be struggling with. It could be the difference between life and death. You're not weak, so don't allow anyone to make you feel that way. Your feelings are valid. Speak up.

chapter 30

Weight Gain / Loss

As explained in the *Healthy Eating* chapter in *Hello, Hello: The Inspirational Guide to Pregnancy* there are ways to help mitigate excessive weight gain during pregnancy. Even while we may do all the right things to reduce weight gain, it's still likely that we will gain something (and most times that is a great sign of a healthy mom and healthy baby). Most moms want to lose the "baby weight" and the truth is that the more we gain the more we will have to work to lose it—unless you were underweight prior to pregnancy or if you just so happen to fall in love with your sexier, curvier, more womanly goddess body (get it hot mama!).

Approximately 60% of moms don't lose the baby weight before our child's first birthday. Therefore, it's more of a normal situation when you still have more weight to lose after year one —meaning you're not alone in your journey. Dropping all of our baby weight immediately after delivery is not only unrealistic for most of us, it's also unnecessary. It's okay to allow yourself time to heal and adjust. The weight loss will come.

Things can change to our bodies post-delivery:

- breasts may get bigger or smaller (droopier if breastfeeding for long periods of time)
- your stomach may never completely flatten (it happens)
- feet may be bigger (time for new shoes)
- hands may be puffier (time for new rings)
- hips may be wider (time for new pants)
- thighs may be thicker (never a bad thing)

Whatever the case, it's all going to be okay. Striving for perfection often isn't the source of inspiration we need. We become our most beautiful selves when we find gratefulness in all that our body was capable of achieving. The more thankful we are, the more humbly we can address our bodies. The more we work to remove those insecurities, the more we can truly learn to love our bodies throughout its entire transition and transformation.

Breastfeeding may or may not speed up weight loss. Every single body is different. Breastfeeding requires your body to produce higher levels of prolactin, which stores excess fat for milk production. This may cause your body to hold on to those last 5-15 pounds that you just can't seem to shake, as it tells your body to hold on to those pounds as fat reserves (should your body need to use those extra reserves to produce milk). Prolactin impacts our body's metabolic activity—slowing it down. So while one mother may just shed pounds while doing nothing, most of us will have to work harder and wait until our breastfeeding journey is over to drop the remaining weight. The truth is the more we stress and obsess over our weight, the more cortisol is released through our body and the harder it will be to lose.

Now is the time to train and brainwash ourselves. We must empower our self perception. You must do what makes you feel beautiful and sexy, even if you have to force yourself into doing it. Find ways to accentuate your new body rather than feeling the need to hide it. People may comment, but the more you rewire your thoughts, the less energy you'll exert into defending your right to look however you please—and the more energy you'll place into the uplift of yourself. You literally just created life. It may take you two months or two years to lose the weight, but you have every right to whatever journey you embark upon.

Humble your expectations. When you feel the need to respond to comments from others, recognize that this may be your ego (puffed up insecurities). We must encourage ourselves and allow our lives to speak volumes—actions are much louder than unnecessary responses or 140 characters. Remember to be thankful and to revitalize your perspective. While you may struggle with an extra couple of pounds, there are women who struggle with the inability to conceive. Remind yourself that there are people all around the world who would give anything to have the opportunity to struggle with baby weight. Strengthen your perspective and have compassion towards yourself. Workout when you can and give yourself time. Find creative ways to work out—even if that includes holding baby while you do so. Stop looking at people online who feel so compelled to show you just how fast they bounced back. Allow your own story to be the dose of inspiration in your life. Permeate your thoughts with humility and gratefulness. Don't ever compare. Just find thankfulness.

this is
your destiny

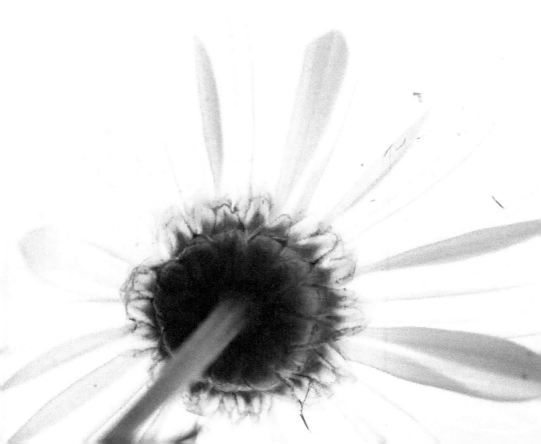

chapter 31

Hair Growth / Loss

Hair loss effects many moms post-delivery. Typically, around 3-6 months postpartum, many see a huge spike in hair loss. This can vary from minimal to drastic. During pregnancy, there was a surge in your estrogen levels. This caused your hair to not only grow faster, but gravely decreased the amount of hair that shed. Post-delivery, your estrogen levels plummet and the hair that was essentially just resting on your head (as it would have normally fallen out without you noticing), will begin to fall out.

If you're someone who experiences the terror of losing chunks of hair, know that it will be okay. It's not permanent and it is completely normal. Around 12 months or so, things should begin to normalize. Try not to stress or panic. There is nothing abnormal about you.

There are remedies you can try to help reduce the amount of hair loss you may experience:

- You can increase your vitamin intake of folic acid, zinc, flaxseeds and vitamins A, C and H.
- Avoid intense styling regiments (i.e. over exposure to heat).
- Avoid over-washing (but remember to keep your hair conditioned and moisturized).

Hair is normally one of the lowest things on our priority list post-delivery and even that is okay. This too (like everything else) is a season. Once you overcome one thing, there will surely be another. You don't have to tackle everything at one time, so decide where your hair is on your priority list and find easy, protective styling options that reduce the amount of effort you have to place into it. You're already supermom whether your hair is long and thick or short and kinky. You got this and you look incredible doing it.

chapter 32

Flight Travel + Outings With Baby

F or many parents, travel with our newborns (and toddlers) are par for the course. Traveling to visit family, enjoying a quick getaway, et cetera, are more common place with babies — even as daunting as travel may seem. Talking with other parents who travel often with babies can be extremely helpful in finding tricks and tips to help make it a smoother occurrence.

Flying is one of the most terrifying things to do with babies (especially long flights). There's an inherent pressure we place on ourselves as parents to ensure our babies are the quietest they've ever been. Not only could it feel embarrassing, but we probably remember the thoughts we harbored about crying babies before we had our own (let's not revisit those). The great news is that, most people are understanding of the hardships of traveling with babies — and they also have headphones, so they won't hear much of it anyway!

The goal is to simply do what you can to keep baby comfortable and surrounded by toys, books, stickers, et cetera, that make the environment identifiable. If and when baby cries (which is more likely to happen as they get older and sleep for shorter periods of time), don't get angry or embarrassed. It happens and the truth is most of us have been there.

There are some ways whereby travel can be less strenuous. Get creative, as every baby is different. Hopefully some of these tips can be of service:

Keep baby hungry for takeoff and landing.

The most important thing to remember is that ear pressure is extremely painful for babies. Often times, if there is a baby who is crying hysterically on a flight with no comfort in sight, it's the pain from the cabin pressure in their ears that is to blame. Unless baby is sleep, it's essential they maintain a sucking pressure (similar to if you were drinking or chewing gum to alleviate pressure in your ears). During the ascent and descent, nurse or bottle feed baby for as long as possible (a slow release nipple may be helpful in elongating the process). If baby doesn't want to eat, or has finished eating, use a soother (pacifier). This will prevent baby's ears from excruciating cabin pressure. Once the plane has made it to its cruising altitude, baby will be just fine.

Bring a stocked snack and activity bag.

Another thing that can make baby antsy is the lack of stimulation. You'll need to keep them entertained — especially as they get older. A newborn (typically starting travel after two months) will sleep for most of the flight. During the remaining time, their favorite activities will be a lifesaver. Pack a bag solely with their favorite books, toys, pacifiers, teething rings, et cetera. Also ensure that you pack enough food and snacks that extend well beyond normal flying time. With unexpected delays and long wait times on tarmacs, you want to ensure that if all else fails, baby will never go hungry during this trip. A hungry baby will be extremely hard to soothe, so pack accordingly — and then add more.

Keep baby warm (get a baby holder).

Most times, baby will want to cuddle and be held by you during flight. Keeping them close to you will not only ward off unwanted touching and germs from strangers, but it will keep them warm. Bringing extra blankets is advisable, as the air is usually blasting on flights. Id it starts to get warm, have lighter clothing options with you as well — to ovoid overheating. Having extra diapers, wipes and clothes is essential, as accidents can happen on flight. A baby holder/carrier may make things easier, as you won't have to physically use your arms to hold them. If they fall asleep in the baby holder, it can be much easier for you to find a comfortable position in your seat. Lastly, bring something clean and warm to place on top of the changing table in the plane bathrooms. They are extremely hard and cold and likely full of germs. Placing something under baby during changing can make them more comfortable and less susceptible to getting sick.

Wait until they have established a routine (and built an immunity).

If you can hold off your travel plans for the first couple of months, it's probably best to do so. Your baby is slowly starting to build their immunity, so the least amount of people they're around, the better. If your flight can't wait — and there are valid reasons why — try to stick to the routine they're starting to establish as best as possible. The more of a routine they have, the calmer they're apt to be.

Choose flights around sleep times, if possible.

Waiting until your newborn has a more predictable sleep schedule can be beneficial for travel as well. If choosing a nighttime flight, get baby dressed in their pajamas and plan for a flight that is around their bedtime (their internal clocks will click in and allow them to sleep — hopefully). Choosing flights around nap time can be a grave help as well, as the goal is to have them sleep as much during flights as possible. The more they sleep, the less you'll have to entertain.

Research to decide if you will hold baby or fly with the car seat.

Most airlines will allow you to hold baby in your lap if they're two years and younger. For some parents, this may make travel easier — especially if you're breastfeeding or you know that they will sleep for most of the flight. For other parents — especially those with multiple children — it may feel safer and less of a hassle to purchase an extra seat on the plane for baby's car seat. This is another way to help establish normalcy for your baby — especially if they're prone to easily fall asleep in their car seat. The choice is completely up to you, so find what works best!

Invest in a stroller cover bag.

As we all know, airline personnel very seldom are careful with our bags. Unfortunately, the same manner by which they tend to carelessly throw luggage, is the same way they may throw your stroller and car seat (which isn't cheap!). Investing in stroller cover bags is a great one, in that they aren't expensive, they fold up really small and can fit in your diaper bag and they will help to avoid unwanted scratches and germs on your baby's car seat and stroller. Most times you'll leave your car seat and stroller at the gate. Having a colored cover bag can make it easier to spot. There are also times when the stroller may be deemed too big and you're then forced to check it. The cover will help to ensure it stays as ding and dirt free as possible. It's definitely worth the investment—especially if you travel often with your little one!

Outings with baby are similar to travel — just less taxing (for the most part). If going to an event with your newborn starts to feel overwhelming, skip it. The more stressed or frazzled you are, the more they will be as well. It doesn't matter what the event is — if you're overwhelmed, it won't be enjoyable. The safety of baby and your sanity comes first in deciding whether to partake in an outing or not.

If an event could negatively impact baby's nap or sleep schedule, more than likely it's more beneficial to skip it — rather than having to start all over in getting the schedule back on track. The truth is people will understand. A baby's schedule is vital to their overall sleep (and yours too!). Your priority is to maintain the schedule you have been working hard to establish, until you notice that baby (possibly when they're a toddler) adjusts well to deviations. If missing a nap ruins the entire day, skip the event. It's probably not worth the melt down. If you can make it and baby can still nap, then do it! You won't have to miss everything, so take advantage of the times when it works out. Occasionally keeping baby out later for events may work for you and if that is the case then great. If you can enjoy time out, you should. It should just never come at the cost of your peace of mind, nor the peace established in your household.

If you're able to enjoy a nice outing with your family, a couple of tips may help make the experience more pleasurable and less stressful:

- **Work around baby's schedule** (sleep comes first). If you have to be a little late or have to leave an event early, that is okay. Do what you can to have as much fun as possible, without throwing baby's schedule out of whack.

- **Have extra snacks and activities on hand** (bringing snacks like shredded cheese, teething crackers, et cetera., can create fun times for baby while you get to actually enjoy some downtime — and possibly a meal!).

- **Bring an extra set of hands if you can.** The more help you have, the less stressful it may be; and the more likely you're to finally enjoy a meal while sitting down.

- **Find family friendly places to go** (kid friendly restaurants, picnics at the park, outings to the museum, are all fun ways to get out of the house and still keep it fun for baby). Space for babies / toddlers to crawl and run is always a great way for them to learn, explore and burn some much needed energy.

- **Do whatever you need to do to keep the stress down.** Essentially, this will involve doing things and bringing foods or activities that create some sense of normalcy and familiarity. The less jarring and shocking for baby, the calmer they will be. Remember to bring things to keep them engaged. The more stimulated they are, the easier it will be for you.

Remember, this is only a season. You must respect where you are and try not to alter or speed it up. In time, things will change and you'll be able to go out significantly more than you do now. But if you worry yourself on making so many events, or if you stress about missing out on so many things, you'll look up to discover that the time has come and gone. You must be present where you are. Before you know it, you'll miss it and wish you took advantage of the time with just you and baby. Prioritize your energy and beware of energy vampires. Follow your mommy gut and simply do you!

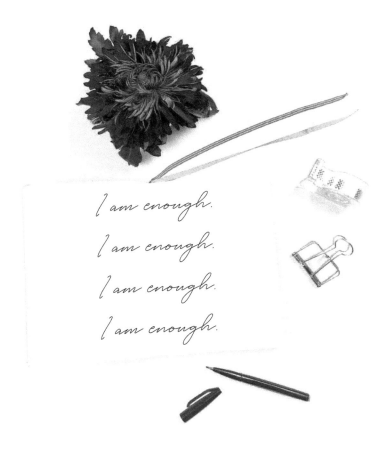

I am enough.
I am enough.
I am enough.
I am enough.

chapter 33

Falling In Love Again (Sex Included)

*I*t's imperative that we honestly address one of the scarier components of postpartum care: losing the spark that created the baby in the first place! Every relationship has different needs—but the goal is to maintain some sort of normalcy for you and your spouse or mate, amidst the grave changes that have and are occurring. The gargantuan shock to the system that happens to moms post-delivery, also happens to dads/partners as well. Though different, it still cannot be minimized or dismissed. This introduction into motherhood is about accepting the evolution of ourselves and our relationships — it's not about completely letting it go to the wayside because of our new livelihood. You must keep the foundation strong and it has to get stronger the harder life gets.

Your baby is coming into YOUR world — you're not changing everything to make it their world.

You and your mate have a rhythm. There are things you love to do and have found to be "your thing" (i.e. Friday night date night). Post baby, many couples tend to throw everything to the side due to the new responsibilities and new schedules. While it's vital to make our babies the priority in our lives, it's even more essential to make the relationship that birthed this baby a priority as well.

You must work together to hold on to those things that make your relationship special and unique. Your baby is coming into your world, so make your schedule work around you and your mate's needs as much as possible. Your baby's schedule should fit into your life in the most ways it can. Obviously, there will be some deviation, but there are still ways to maintain some familiarity of your world. If this requires baby's schedule being more flexible or more rigid, you and your mate will know what that is. It may take some time and lots of trial and error, but you and your mate must be a priority.

If, for example, Friday night was date night prior to baby, you should try and maintain it as much as you can. If this means every other Friday, or the first Friday of every month, you must make it a priority the same way you make baby's sleeping schedule a priority. Your relationship cannot become an afterthought. It has to be the first thought, because if the relationship goes, parenting will get exponentially harder.

You must find things that connect you both to what made you fall in love in the first place, but allows that love to evolve, grow and deepen. It's those unique and quirky things that keep you from simply being roommates or just best friends. Deciding to keep your relationship a priority is not selfish — but a necessity. Understanding that you must heed to the needs of your partner is essential to a thriving relationship with such a drastic change in it. Both of you will be exhausted, irritable, confused, happy, et cetera. You'll feel a range of emotions and often times they won't be at the same time. Focusing on keeping each other happy is vital, because if the sole focus is on baby, you'll start to move apart from each other. If you and your mate focus on each other, you'll be surprised at how fulfilling parenting will be together.

You and your spouse/partner come first.

Whether it sounds selfish or feels wrong, the truth is, it's not! Most times we neglect everything and everybody for the sake of our baby. Though innate, we must put work in to ensure we have enough energy to care for and love hard on our mate as well. Though it may take some time (and that is perfectly normal, especially with a baby tugging at your nipples for 18 hours a day), it's still worth the work and definitely worth paying attention to.

You must come first to each other. This will help to ensure a solid foundation by which all of the hardships fall — and it helps to develop and maintain strong communication (and more listening). The more you put the needs of your spouse/partner first, the more you can and will listen without judgment. The more you can find understanding in each others emotions and hard times and the more you'll choose to ask for help before assuming the worst in each other. A lot gets lost in translation;

especially when everyone is sleep deprived. When we can honor our partnerships and place it at the forefront of all we do, nothing (not even sleep deprivation) can break it apart.

It's also worth noting that in 18 years (maybe more, but who's counting), when baby is grown and ready to explore the world away from home, it will be back to you and your mate. The more you put your relationship first — refusing to allow baby / children to cause riffs or dissent — the stronger it will be when the next huge transition comes. Putting yourselves first does NOT equate to neglect of your child(ren), rather the opposite. about refusing to neglect your love of each other, in hopes of creating and establishing a stronger foundation whereby to raise your babies. You'll be their example of unconditional love.

You must frequently date (preferably within the first month).

You MUST do baby free things. This is key. You must try and keep things as nuanced as possible — which will be extremely hard to do within this first year. Getting stuck in a monotonous routine without any excitement, is a huge component that leads to resentment, lack of communication, depression and feeling alone and isolated. Our spouses will not know exactly how we as mom feel all the time and we shouldn't expect them to. But the more you can go out, have fun and love on each other, the more time you'll have to discover and rediscover one another. From this foundation, you'll find more compassionate communication, father than resentful and angry.

Not having any nuanced experiences (especially with your mate) fundamentally goes against how we were designed by nature. Once our routine becomes stagnant and predictable, we lose a sense of who we are — and that is because we are creatures of creativity and new experiences. Going out on a date is more than just dating at this phase of life — is it the start to falling in love with this new place you're in together. This is how you recreate and reimagine who you are as a couple and it's how you start the process of loving on each other, baby free!

Communication is more pivotal now than ever before.

Keeping your thoughts and feelings inside is a recipe for animosity and assumption. During this time, someone (usually mom) will always feel they're doing more work than the other. Moms tend to feel extremely isolated (less freedom, always tied down to nursing), especially while dad/partner gets to go out and back to work like nothing ever happened. It's way too easy to fall into a space of jealously and resentment of our mate's freedom. Their normalcy is infuriating if we don't feel appreciated or understood.

Hence, the importance of being open and honest. In your open communication (always talk to your mate before you talk to other people about your problems), you may discover pains you never knew existed — especially when you're in a safe relationship. In talking with your mate, you may discover that while you resent their ability to leave and go to work, they may resent the fact you get to spend so much quality time with baby. They may feel like a stranger, out of place and always messing up the routine. Most people want what they don't have and are jealous about fairy tale scenarios that don't really exist.

We must always assume positive intent with our mate. Tell them when you feel overwhelmed — don't let it fester and build up internally. You'll implode and at that point it gets harder to discover the true issue you're dealing with. It may actually be a lack of sleep, rather than feeling unloved from your spouse. It may actually be a lack of help, rather than believing your mate is out partying at work while you're struggling at home. Find understanding through your communication and practice patience with one another. You're both on a learning curve — so offer the same patience and compassion that you require. Be open to each other's differences and don't judge the varied approaches. You both are different, so expect nuanced parenting styles. Find the space that cohesively fuses the two styles together and be okay with what you both create. If baby feels loved, then all is well (plus, you can re-do the diaper later when he's not looking).

Don't allow yourself the space and opportunity to feel alone — especially when your mate is right there. If you're angry, strive to find calmness and humility prior to speaking. Choose to speak with love, because at the end of the day, love is the best choice. Try to remember you're both exhausted, which often times exacerbates the situation. Don't give up on each other, because you two come first. The spark will come back. Be open, be honest, give yourself time and speak with love. You'll be surprised at how willing they are to help you in any way possible. Just ask (kindly).

Be open and honest about your feelings towards sex.

Remember that during breastfeeding, your body releases oxytocin and has lower levels of estrogen which decreases your sex drive. It's important to understand what your body is going through so you can cut yourself some slack. The hard part is not allowing those changes to become the new norm in your house.

It can be extremely hard to find any sort of desire to have sex post-delivery. The exhaustion alone is enough to make you feel like all you ever want to do is close your eyes when you lay down at night. Sometimes getting in the mood for sex can feel like work (sometimes it is). This is why it's important to be honest with each other, because the last thing you ever want is for the love of your life to feel rejected. If them taking on more responsibility means more energy for you, they may surprise you with all they'll do to make that happen!

If you're nursing, remember your oils! Low levels of estrogen reduces your vaginal mucous — so you'll be dry down there. Dress sexy on occasion and try different tactics that can start to bring back your interest — not for your partner but for you. You must allow yourself the space to feel beautiful and sexy again. Speaking openly about your feelings may be all you need to get things going. The great news is that in time, your sex drive will return. This also goes back to the importance of dating. Do what makes you both feel sexy and get rid of the notion of "mom clothes". Being a mom does not equate to dressing dull or wearing oversized clothing all of a sudden. You don't have to change your eccentric and fly style because you're a mom. Love yourself on this journey and don't let go. Don't lose sight of who your mate fell in love with and they won't either.

Before things get really exciting again, be sure to also openly communicate about contraceptives. Discuss during pregnancy or during the recovery phase of postpartum care (the six weeks of no sex), ways that you both will focus on pregnancy prevention — if that's your goal. This is important because that surprise pregnancy is always just one fun night away!

Do things that make you both feel normal.

You must fall in love with your newly evolved self in order to fall harder in love with your mate. Your relationship will be different and understanding and accepting that will make the transition much more harmonious. Don't expect everything to be the same — that just isn't realistic. But don't give up on each other because things are different — that isn't efficient or effective. It's about exploring together to find your new space as one. In time, you'll find it only gets stronger and the love gets more intense with each sleepless night. And remember, however you go into parenthood is how it will be. Whatever you decide it will be, it will be. So speak powerfully over your new journey. If you say things won't be easy, they won't be. If you say this will be the greatest journey you both have ever embarked on, it will be. Decide what you both want and go get it.

Kiss, hug and say I love you all the time.

These intimacies plus sex are the only things that truly separate our spouse or partner from everyone else. They are the things that distinguish between having a best friend or roommate and having a life partner. As simple as it may seem, kissing often during your postpartum healing can go a long way. You want to avoid creating new norms or habits of constantly needing space — and never seeking or giving intimacy. In your new normal, intimacy and romance must be part of the equation.

Becoming a mom doesn't equate to giving up on the romance or the sexy (maternity clothes will need to go at some point). The truth is that most days, you'll be in your comfy sweats and leggings, raggedy shirts, bandanas, et cetera. When you don't feel sexy, you probably won't act that way towards your spouse either. Again, that is okay. You aren't required to be in the mood or get them in the mood at all times. But there are times when we should. Every now and again, we must allow ourselves the time and space to feel sexy and free (whatever that means for you — if that means mom jeans and maternity leggings, then get it in!). Not only will we feel good, but your mate will love it as well.

When the times arise that you're just too tired to engage, share how you feel and don't forget to kiss and hug. The goal is to maintain intimacy and romance the best way possible — because it's a vital component in the fabric of your relationship. Find ways to have fun when baby goes to sleep. Remember that intimacy and romance does not have to be reserved for night. Be adventurous and love hard. And say I love you every single day. You'll need it and so do they.

Laugh.

Laugh just because! You're in this thing together and there is no turning back. There will be some things you just can't do anything about (i.e. your little one waking up four times a night due to teething). In those times, don't give in to the anger. This will require work, but we are capable of putting in that work. Not only are we capable, but we need to in order to maintain sanity and peace. Find something to laugh about every day. Make it a requirement — soon it may become second nature.

Before bed, every night, do or say something to make each other smile and/or laugh. It's the only way to keep you both at peace with each other. Our brains don't know the difference between a fake laugh or a real one, but what's true is that whenever you smile or laugh, oxytocin is released through your body. The more you tell yourself that you feel good (even if forced), the more you'll actually feel good. The more you feel good, the better your thoughts. The better your thoughts, the better you can handle the tough moments. The more tough moments you overcome, the stronger your relationship. The stronger your relationship, the harder you'll love. And the harder you love, the more impenetrable the relationship becomes — meaning, no one, no circumstance, no single thing can break what you have.

Say I love you and don't take each other for granted. You create your fairytale. Be kind. And be love for each other.

Focus on sex post baby (it is important).

It's important to give yourself time to adjust to your new body and your new life. But no matter what, you must make it a point to fall in love with sex with your spouse/partner.

Sex post-delivery can be scary at first, so when it's time, go slow. Take your time and remember your oils (coconut, aloe, et cetera). Remember to take it easy and be aware of your body. You may bleed a little after the first couple of times, which is normal. Don't downplay the impact foreplay can have as you get back into the swing of things. You may need a little extra time and work to finally get into the mood, especially while mother nature is working against your libido. Hopefully, as you get into the mood, it will become fun and liberating for you.

Things don't have to take three hours either (to be honest, you'll probably be up with baby in three hours). Just be in the moment and enjoy. Don't get in the habit of perpetually thinking about it "being over with". Your spouse will feel that and it could possibly feel like rejection.

Post-delivery, most moms are acutely more aware of our bodies. Use this to your advantage. Listen to your body and speak up. It may be hard to get into the groove, but more often than not, you'll be happy you did. Sex is not only important for maintaining the spark, but it's also a great stress reliever for you as well (and a workout). The goal is simply to give yourself time to fall back in love with sex and to avoid creating a new norm of little to no sex with your spouse/partner. Love on each other — and if you need more help, work together to find ways to evolve and grow. Sex is important, so treat it as such.

chapter 34

Opinions of Others (Feeling Judged)

*O*pinions of others seem almost impossible to avoid. Hopefully the following will help you navigate your way through negative spaces (even those that are well intentioned). Take what works and ignore what doesn't.

You probably won't ask for most of the advice given to you.

When someone offers their awesome parenting advice, it may be to combat whatever you're currently doing, or out of sheer excitement for your journey. Whatever the case, many times the first instinct is to defend ourselves. Fortunately, you don't have to explain or defend yourself to anyone. Online, you don't have to share everything you do — helping to avoid creating a space whereby people can comment and share their opinions. Don't put yourself in a position or around people you know will make you feel inadequate as a mother (you know who and what these are). Protect your heart and keep in mind how sensitive this time is (even though others might not).

Try to assume positive intent rather than assuming the worst. Try not to get offended by the opinions of others — if it works for you take it, if it doesn't, keep it pushing. Feel free to let people know you're good to go — or simply say thank you. The less energy you give to others, the more you'll have for yourself and baby. The less thought you give to it, the less likely it can negatively impact your day.

You know your baby best.

Your mommy gut is strong, so trust it and listen to your intuition. In the same breath, be open to advice from others — but be careful with whom you confide in. Guard your heart and again, beware of those energy vampires who are known to suck anything good from the room. Choose your circle and your support system wisely. It will likely be bigger or smaller than you think. And remember people who don't have babies can only intellectualize what you're going through but so much. There is something extremely unique and nuanced about parenthood and it's unlike anything else in life. Don't get upset if your childfree friends or family members don't understand. They are truly incapable of completely understanding. Find those who have been through or are going through what you are. Empathy is essential — and talking with other parents will offer you wisdom that is unmatched!

Talk to your spouse/partner 1st (before anyone else).

Always confide in your spouse/partner first! Work things out together first. Keep things at home and remember to respect one another. Stay out of other people's business and keep people out of yours. Figure out what works best for your relationship. Be open to allowing change and be flexible with your newly evolved space. Set your foundation tougher and make conscious decisions together on what you both are unwilling to waiver on and what you're open to changing. You two come first. Always.

Mom-shammers are simply deflecting their own insecurities onto you (don't fall for it).

Any mom who can speak negatively about another mom is completely dishonest with herself. A person who can verbally assault and shame someone else who is trying to do their very best, is likely unhappy and insecure about her own abilities as a mother (don't let the ego fool you). Don't appease anyone's insecurities with a response. Your response back often times doesn't prove anything other than you are indeed willing to engage. Don't employ yourself in the convincing business. Mind your family and mind your business. Their useless and weightless words are not your business and unworthy of a response.

Don't let any outside forces interrupt the peace within your home and your family. And don't let your own insecurities or ego cause you to respond negatively towards anyone else. You don't have to explain your choices to anyone—and no one has to explain their choices to you. Your decisions to use pacifiers for three months or three years, to start potty training at 15 or 36 months, putting your babies to bed late or early, allowing them to drink juice or not, choosing formula over nursing, et cetera — whatever it is, it's your decision. Your family deserves your energy and with love at the foundation, there is simply no room for anything or anyone else.

Trust and believe that you can be a great mother.

No single person on this planet has cracked the code to parenting. It constantly evolves and culturally we are becoming more open to the notion that every child is indeed different. We're all just figuring this parenting thing out as we go — even the moms online who have all the answers when it comes to your choices. Follow your heart and your gut. Use wisdom from those whose parenting has inspired you. Be open to learning and learn all you can from those who have been there. Wisdom is simply semantic knowledge coupled with experiential knowledge. Talk to older parents to get some wisdom on their experiences and talk with younger parents who are in the thick of things with you. Remain open, but don't allow yourself the opportunity to be judged. There is no competition and you're not in a race. Just take it one day at a time.

Your primary goal as a parent is to instill the best foundation for your children to go out and thrive in the world. Doing your best requires being your best — and that requires respecting yourself and loving your journey. Find joy in everything and if anyone or anything strips away that joy, let it go. Let it go. Let it go.

If you feel like giving up, remember how lucky you are.

There is a beautiful young woman I know who had an extremely tumultuous pregnancy. She was chronically ill and had to get tests done for herself and her baby the entire 9 months. Through her fears, feeling as if her body had failed her and the sheer terror of simply throwing a baby shower, she pushed on regardless. This incredible mom birthed her baby, who suffered from a rare heart condition. She and her husband spent six days with their newborn before he gained his angel wings. She went through pregnancy, delivery, and the postpartum phase to only have six short days with her baby. Even after the six days, her body still acted as if her angel was with her. Imagine having to endure all of the postpartum effects without being able to kiss your baby every morning or rocking them in the middle of the night when they don't feel well. Imagine not being able to do all of the things that make us frustrated. Imagine this mom and imagine what she would give to struggle the way you get to with your baby. Imagine what she would give to smell her baby's scent just one more time. Imagine her and imagine the thousands of other moms who are experiencing the same thing as we speak.

Sometimes it's important to simply reflect on how blessed we truly are. We must take the time to notice that there are people right now who would give anything to be right where you are. A shift in perspective doesn't minimize how hard motherhood is. It's simply a source of inspiration that we must inject ourselves with, in order to encourage ourselves to never give up. We must keep on going and we must remind ourselves that we can and will make it through the hard times. Just remember how blessed you are to even get to experience these hard times. For they are the very things making you a better, stronger, more empowered light being on this earth.

You are still your biggest critic.

No one will be harder on you then you. You must be kind to yourself. Stop judging and being so hard on yourself, and stop expecting perfection. Remember your worth and be open to change. The more you embrace change, the easier the process will become. Be open to receiving help. Listen and trust yourself. Beware those energy vampires — and be aware if you are one yourself. Do whatever you need in order to find peace. Breathe. Meditate. Write. Exercise. Sit still, or get wild. Remember that you were built for this. Look at your body and remember that baby chose your body to be brought into this life to change the world. This was no mistake. This is your destiny.

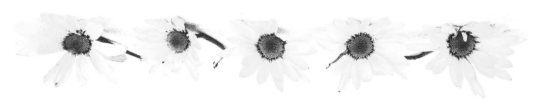

You Are Everything

T here is so much that goes on during this first year of motherhood (and every year afterwards). It's a never-ending journey. So be excited and proud of yourself for wherever you are. The entire purpose of *Hello, Hello: The Inspirational Guide to Pregnancy, Delivery, and PostPartum* was purely to encourage you through your journey, and provide you the basic information you'll need for the start of your own research. I tried to tackle as many topics as I could, with as much sensitivity, openness, and kindness as possible. My goal has been to ignite your curiosity about this journey into motherhood, spark your desire to learn more, and remind you that you're never alone.

Parenting is personal. No one can tell you what to do. But the more you equip yourself with the knowledge and education you need, the less you can be manipulated into doing anything that feels contrary to who you are and what you believe. Find moments of stillness amidst the nonstop chaos — and in that stillness, listen to your heart.

This book series was designed to inspire more confidence in yourself and your capabilities. Things will get messy and sometimes complicated. There may be times where you question yourself and everything you're doing. But at the end of the day, it's all good.

It's how you go into your journey that will set you apart from even your greatest fears. It's about how you direct your energy and where you choose to place your habitual thoughts. Don't focus on the struggle and don't fight against the things you don't want. Don't become paralyzed by fear or anxiety. Simply focus on what you want. Whatever you say will be. If you say it will be hard, it will be. If you have empowered thoughts, your journey will reflect that. Focus on what you want exclusively, and watch how the universe grants those desires to you.

Hone in on your dreams and never stop dreaming. Becoming a mother is not now, nor will it ever be, the deterrent to your hopes and visions. You're not *just a mom*. You're a light being with a mission to bring about change to this world through your life and the lives of the child(ren) you bring up. Never limit your capabilities. You can become all of the things you dream of with a bit of sacrifice, patience, and empathy for yourself.

Love harder than you ever have before — and exemplify that love for your child(ren). Don't give in to your exhaustion, and believe every day that you'll make it through this moment.

When you love who you are, everything changes.

Your truth will be magnified through motherhood, so it's imperative that at the start, you're honest with yourself — finding honesty in the things that serve you and letting go of all that does not. Once you find the openness and compassion for accepting everything about yourself, then move forward. Don't dwell in the past. Exert energy into this most precious time you have, right now. Honor your journey, and respect yourself and your spouse/partner.

Believe and accept that you're a goddess.

You're the creator of life and the foundation whereby baby will view the world and their possibilities. Honor your child(ren)'s innocence. They will believe whatever you tell them.

Words mean what they mean — choose wisely.

Embrace the journey and love it.

Choose love, for love is a choice.

Remember how beautiful the world is. Travel, explore, and learn together as a family. You're not here by accident and you were not created to just take up space. The universe chose you — don't deny that power. Your baby chose you — don't ignore the significance of their choice. Honor your gift with everything you have and nurture all the possibilities life has to offer.

I hope you are as inspired by this read as I am by you.

You're a light being before all other labels, and when you choose to let it shine, there is no denying just how powerful you are. Allow your light to shine the brightest it ever has before. You'll make it through.

So smile.

For the truth of the matter is that, you already have.

From my heart to yours, with love from the depths of my soul. See you on the journey ;)

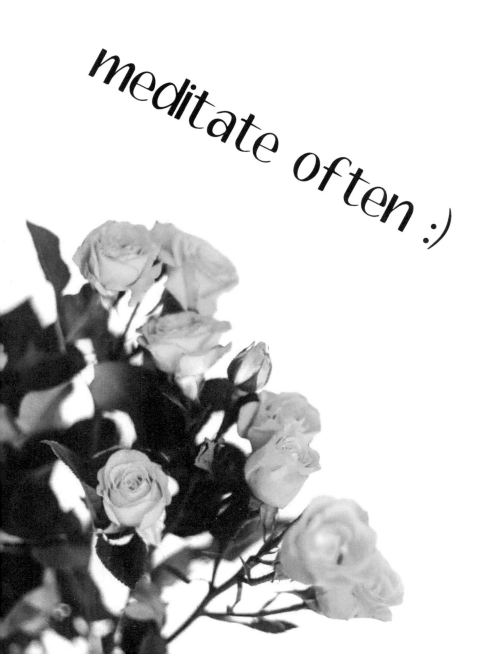

meditate often :)

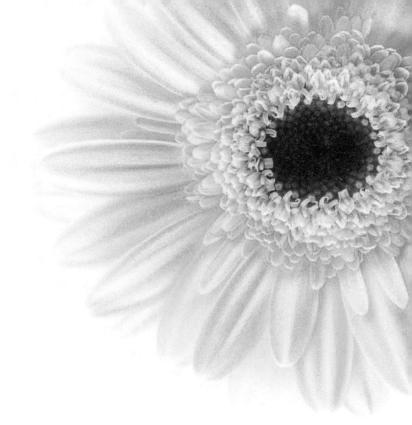

May
this land
exactly where
it needs to.

Endnotes

[1] Reproductive Health. (2018, May 09). Retrieved September, 2018, from https://www.cdc.gov/reproductivehealth/maternalinfanthealth/pregnancy-relatedmortality.htm

[2] Martin, P. N., & Montagne, R. (2017, May 12). U.S. Has The Worst Rate Of Maternal Deaths In The Developed World. Retrieved September, 2018, from https://www.npr.org/2017/05/12/528098789/u-s-has-the-worst-rate-of-maternal-deaths-in-the-developed-world

[3] High-Risk Pregnancy. (n.d.). Retrieved December, 2018, from https://www.ucsfhealth.org/conditions/high-risk_pregnancy/

[4] Wallerstein, E. (1983). The Circumcision Decision. *International Childbirth Education Association.*

[5] WhattoExpect. (2018, December 18). 6 Tips to Care for Your Newborn's Umbilical Cord. Retrieved May, 2018, from https://www.whattoexpect.com/baby-growth/umbilical-cord-care.aspx

[6] Pearson-Glaze, P. (2018, July 04). No Breast Milk After Delivery. Retrieved August, 2018, from https://breastfeeding.support/no-breast-milk-after-delivery/

[7] Malachi, R. (2018, December 11). 8 Practical Ways New Moms Can Deal With Postpartum Insomnia. Retrieved January, 2019, from https://www.momjunction.com/articles/tips-to-handle-postnatal-insomnia_00329713/#gref

[8] Malachi, R. (2018, December 11).

[9] Domas, K. (2018, February 20). How Does Stress Impact Breastfeeding? Retrieved January, 2019, from https://insured.amedadirect.com/stress-impact-breastfeeding/

[10] The National Institute of Mental Health Information Resource Center. (n.d.). Postpartum Depression Facts. Retrieved June, 2018, from https://www.nimh.nih.gov/health/publications/postpartum-depression-facts/index.shtml

[11] Baylor University. (2016, June 23). United States parents not as happy as those without children, researcher says. *ScienceDaily*. Retrieved August 30, 2019 from www.sciencedaily.com/releases/2016/06/160623065405.htm

[12] Babbel, S. (2010, December 8). Postpartum PTSD Versus Postpartum Depression. Retrieved September, 2018, from https://www.psychologytoday.com/us/blog/somatic-psychology/201012/postpartum-ptsd-versus-postpartum-depression

[13] Fisher, S. P. (2017, September 7). Traumatic Deliveries. Retrieved September, 2018, from https://www.psychologytoday.com/us/blog/beyond-the-egg-timer/201709/traumatic-deliveries

[14] Reinberg, S. (2019, March 11). SIDS Risk Doubles If Mom Smoked in Pregnancy. Retrieved from https://www.webmd.com/parenting/news/20190311/sids-risk-doubles-if-mom-smoked-in-pregnancy#1

[15] BabyCenter, & BabyCenter Medical Advisory Board. (2017, October). Postpartum urinary incontinence. Retrieved December, 2018, from https://www.babycenter.com/0_postpartum-urinary-incontinence_1152241.bc

Meet the Author

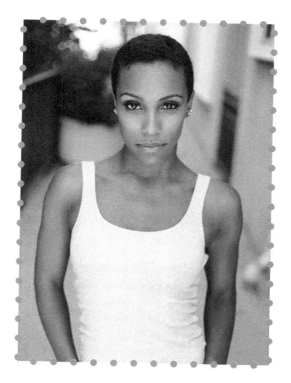

*T*he accomplishments set forth by Danielle Jai Watson are to be revered with this young philanthropic artist. Post-graduation from Pepperdine University, she immediately began working professionally in the entertainment industry; dancing and performing nationally and internationally with world renowned artists including but not limited to Usher, Beyonce, Pharrell, Will I Am, Justin Bieber, Nicki Minaj, Nicole Scherzinger, Shakira and Mariah Carey.

Most notably, she has trained, worked with and been mentored by the legendary Debbie Allen. Offered a complete scholarship to the Debbie Allen Dance Academy, Danielle trained with Ms. Allen full time, while also attending school full time at Pepperdine University; graduating in three years with a degree in Integrated Marketing Communications, and a minor focus in International Business and Grant Writing for non-profits. She attributes much of her success in school and dance to the guidance and support of not only her extraordinarily inspiring family, but the discipline and unparalleled focus she gained being a mentee of Ms. Allen's.

While at the peak of her career, Danielle, alongside husband Dion Watson, engaged full time into their youth performing arts program in Compton, CA, Discover.YOU™, Inc. Focused on providing Performing and Liberal Arts classes, tutoring, and mentorship opportunities to the youth in the community, they taught free dance and choreography workshops to local youth. Soon thereafter, they opened the doors to their very own facility in Compton, CA, where they ran their extended programming to youth — all on full scholarships.

She continues to pursue her passion and sincere love for the arts. In 2016, she and her husband welcomed their son King Jay Watson and, fifteen months later, daughter Zenzile Monét Louise Watson. After having two empowered medically-free vaginal births, she began mentoring young women who were embarking on their pregnancy, delivery, and postpartum journeys. Her passion and personal journey of helping the greater community led her to write three books: *Hello, Hello: The Inspirational Guide to* **Pregnancy**; *Hello, Hello: The Inspirational Guide to* **Delivery**; and *Hello, Hello: The Inspirational Guide to* **Postpartum**.

With a mission to empower the greater community, that is exactly what Danielle plans to do. A light being, wife, mother, dreamer, writer, creative, dancer, mentor and philanthropist, the best is truly yet to come.

Lightning Source UK Ltd.
Milton Keynes UK
UKHW050654120620
364766UK00007B/53